A Country Doctor's Chronicle

A Country Doctor's Chronicle

FURTHER TALES FROM THE NORTH WOODS

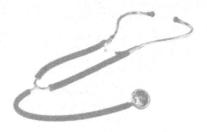

Roger A. MacDonald, MD

BOREALIS
BOOKS

BOREALIS BOOKS is an imprint of the Minnesota Historical Society Press.

www.borealisbooks.org

The Minnesota Historical Society Press is a member of the Association of American University Presses.

Manufactured in the United States of America

10 9 8 7 6 5 4 3 2 1

∞ The paper used in this publication meets the minimum requirements of the American National Standard for Information Sciences—Permanence for Printed Library materials, ANSI Z39.48-1984.

International Standard Book Number 0-87351-509-9 (cloth)

Library of Congress Cataloging-in-Publication Data

MacDonald, Roger A., 1924–

A country doctor's chronicle : further tales from the north woods / Roger A. MacDonald.

    p. ; cm.

Sequel to: A country doctor's casebook. c2002.

ISBN 987-1-68134-023-4 (casebound : alk. paper)

1. MacDonald, Roger A., 1924–
2. Physicians—Minnesota—Biography.
3. Medicine, Rural—Minnesota.

[DNLM: 1. MacDonald, Roger Allen, 1924– 2. Physicians—Minnesota—Personal Narratives. 3. Rural Health Services—Minnesota—Personal Narratives. WZ 100 M137c 2004]
I. MacDonald, Roger A., 1924– Country doctor's casebook. II. Title.

R154.M15A3 2004

610'.92—dc22

2004008630

A Country Doctor's Chronicle

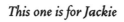

This one is for Jackie

Introduction

I HAVE BEEN extraordinarily fortunate, and in so many ways: the joys and support of family; professional challenges, opportunities, and adventures; the chance to live in an area I love, among people I like and respect; a taste of what pioneer ancestors sought, independence to make my own decisions; a knowledge, day by day, that my work was needed and appreciated.

Beginning in 1948 and for much of the next forty-six years, I was a country doctor in that part of northern Minnesota which was last to be settled. In the earliest years of the twentieth century, a handful of Euro-Americans "founded" the village where I began my practice. Several of them were still alive when I arrived, and I reveled in listening to their tales, history vibrant on their lips.

Because a family doctor is central to the medical care provided in an isolated community, she or he becomes intimately involved in the townspeople's lives. Patients become friends, and friends become patients. To know each patient as a person, not as merely a name or a file number, is the privilege of a country doctor. A physician accumulates a host of stories over the span of a career: people hurting, laughing, living, dying, loving, and procreating. So many confidences must go with the doctor to his or her grave, yet the urge to share examples of human courage and resourcefulness clamors for expression.

My deceased first wife, Barbara, was a registered nurse. We worked together, and our kids grew up hearing us rehash the day's events over the supper table. "Dad, write down your stories," they said. Ja sure, someday.

I worked for the University of Minnesota Medical School in Minneapolis during the final decade of my career. To demonstrate the joys of rural practice, the university placed third-year medical students in the offices of select small-town physicians. I traveled all over the state, visiting rural clinics and hospitals. As I worked with these bright, idealistic youths, I recounted anonymous tales from my "pioneer" experiences. "Write them down!" many said. Ja sure, someday.

A historian recording early happenings in my part of northern Minnesota contacted me for a short essay about "the old days in medicine." I obliged. "Write down those stories," she said. Ja sure, someday.

Someday arrived. The result was *A Country Doctor's Casebook: Tales from the North Woods*, published in 2002 by Borealis Books. The chief hurdle I had to clear in writing that book involved maintaining my patients' confidentiality. Telling the stories was easy; disguising identities required more effort. All of the stories in that book, as in this one, relate actual happenings. Nevertheless, I frequently altered extraneous details in order to conceal identities.

Facing the same dilemma of confidentiality with this collection, I followed two options. When ongoing personal contact allowed, I obtained permission from the patient to use his or her story. In other cases—the majority, as most of these events occurred decades ago—I altered identifying details, retaining the essence of the story, the glimpse of human character, or I combined several similar events and invented a single character. In all cases involving patients, I have used fictitious names. And, of course, opinions expressed in what follows are those of the author.

The publication of *A Country Doctor's Casebook* yielded a round of book signings across Minnesota and Wisconsin. At these readings I encountered former patients; medical-school classmates not seen for fifty years; old friends from venues as varied as the softball field behind the Littlefork Catholic church and scattered small towns such as Northome, "The Falls," Grand Rapids, Hibbing, St. Peter, and Montevideo; colleagues who had also lived through the medical adventures of an isolated practice; and students I had been privileged to supervise, now emerged from the chrysalis of medical education unscathed, performing with confidence and skill. There were:

Mike, son of good friend Ira, Nett Lake Chippewa Reservation Indian agent, grown from a lively lad into a staid grandpa.

Littlefork neighbors who had shared canasta and charades and square dancing to while away those long winter evenings fifty years ago, when thirty degrees below zero was the norm.

Dr. John Menefee, friend of sixty years, a dentist who provided his skill where really needed. I remind him: "We were fishing and you were trying to remove a hook from the mouth of an annoyed northern pike. You muttered, in the conditioned reflex of the profession, 'Wider, please.'"

Effie Hanover, widow of Dr. Ralph Hanover, my first practice mentor. Frail as are most in their nineties, but with sparkle intact.

Mrs. T. sits beside the table to have her book signed. Her

smiles belie the lines hard work and climate have etched on her cheeks. "Doctor, you delivered six of my children," she says. "One time we just didn't have the money to pay you for the last baby, but I was expecting again. You told me to forget it, that we'd start over." She opens her purse. "Doctor, I can pay you now." I develop an acute case of the sniffles.

A man grins at me from across the table. Yes, Oscar, I recall you well—and fondly.

A matronly lady says, "Remember me? You delivered me." My standard response to such an announcement has become, "You've changed." Sitting beside me, my wife, Jackie, turns red to keep from laughing.

A lady pushes her book across the table to be signed—and begins to cry. I had last worked in her town fifty years before, and she was clearly younger than that. "My dad," she manages. "He fell onto the whirling blade of a great circular saw in a mill, chopping his arm to pieces. He always said you saved it for him." Gulp.

In Northome, we share a meal with Dr. Gordon Franklin and wife Midge, registered nurse and office partner. For half a century they have devoted their lives to providing care to members of their community. Shared tales, shared memories, shared understanding award those who have walked the same road. Love and respect seal a friendship.

In the past, I used the name "Northpine" to represent all the communities in which I have worked. For this book, I have decided to continue that practice. However, as I have also chosen to address some issues that are more generic but personally important, I will at times place people and locales with better accuracy.

I offer these further stories with the hope, first, that I offend no one and, second, that the blessings and trust given me by so many over the years might illuminate a problem or offer inspiration to someone traveling a dark and lonely road.

Decades after the event, fact can yield to wishful recollection. I am indebted to Ms. Lee Heffron and Bob VonAlman for helping keep memories of those long-ago days on track and to Ms. Eleanor Waha, Ms. Mildred Thoreson, and Ms. Rosemary Lamson, RN, for improving the accuracy of the chapter "Where There's the Will."

Can an author arrive at a finished product without the benevolent guidance of a good editor? Has any author had a more understanding guide than I? Thank you again, Ms. Shannon Pennefeather.

As I have noted elsewhere, there is a marvelous egalitarianism among rural Minnesotans. Deeds and character earn respect; titles tend to be tolerated rather than revered. While a few locals persisted in addressing me as "Doctor," most quickly adopted "Roger" or my initials, "RAM." If decorum dictated formality, I became "Doc." Mutual regard was never a casualty.

A Country Doctor's Chronicle

House Calls

DURING MY TRAVELS in behalf of *A Country Doctor's Casebook*, the question I was asked most often was some variation of "Did you *really* make house calls?"

Yes, Virginia, I frequently made house calls.

I understand that it is more efficient for a patient to come to the doctor. It is difficult to take an x-ray in a Cingmars Township farmhouse, and, when the nearest drugstore is fifty miles away, what does one do if Mrs. Smith needs cephalexin more than the aspirin on hand? Still, seeing people in their own surroundings helped me understand stresses in their lives that might have been incomprehensible otherwise, and I did not begrudge most house calls.

Oh, there were occasions.

One cold winter's night I awoke to the clamor of my bedside telephone. I squinted at the clock: 3:30 AM. I muttered a greeting into the mouthpiece of the instrument cradled beside my pillow.

I heard, "Doc MacDonald?"

"Yes?"

"You gotta come out here right away."

"Where is 'here'?" I yawned.

"Our house!"

"Where is our house? That is, your—"

"Craigville!"

(He must be kidding. Sixty miles away, and no one lives in Craigville any—)

"No one lives out there anymore."

"We do! Maggie an' me."

(Surely the guy's name can't be Jiggs. Tricks the half-asleep mind plays.)

I mumbled, "Jiggs who? That is—Sir, who are you?"

"Maggie's husband! What's with the Jiggs crap?"

I was beginning to keep one eye propped open. The clock reported the birth of another minute . . . or its death.

(Profound philosophical dilemma there.)

"Sorry." Really deep yawn. "Maggie's Husband," I said, "what seems to be wrong with you?"

"Me? Nothin'! Aren't you listening?"

"Maybe I dozed off. Who's sick with what?"

"How do I know? That's what you docs is for."

My wife, Barbara, poked me in the back, a signal to get up or shut up. "Sir," I said firmly, "what *exactly* is your problem?"

Maggie's associate said, "The old lady's been yammerin' at me for six months she don't feel good. I'm sick of hearin' about it, and I want you to come on out and find what's the matter."

I hung up the receiver and snuggled close to the lovely not-Maggie beside me.

. . .

During the early days of my practice, I still considered a request for a house call to be a command. It had not occurred to me that any remotely reasonable-sounding appeal might be denied.

One day Josh Thompson called. "Doc, ya need to come on out our farm."

"What's the matter?"

"Nellie's got herself the flu."

"Can you bring her in?"

"Hell, Doc, I told ya, she's got the flu."

"Well, okay. Where?"

"We-uns live eighteen miles out the Hardscrabble Road, second driveway past the Dew Drop Inn Tavern. When ya comin'?"

"Say five, five-thirty; after office hours."

"That late? She don't feel so good. Oh, since you're comin' anyhow, stop by Meinert's Market an' pick up our grocery order. They close at five-thirty, so you don't wanna mess up."

"I beg your—"

Dial tone.

I picked up Thompson's grocery order, including a thirty-pound bag of dog food. When I arrived, I had to wait while flu-ravaged Nellie finished milking the cows, her husband having disappeared on some obscure mission.

"Have to send us a bill, Doc," Nellie said, "'counta Josh, he's got the checkbook."

A week later, Rob Stacy stopped me on the street. "Doc, that trip to Thompson's? I happened to be there when he called you. I said something about it being pretty cheeky, asking you to bring the groceries, said you should charge him double. Josh told me, 'Hell, I ain't goin' pay that rich S.O.B. *anything*.'"

I never again delivered groceries.

.   .   .

So, house calls. Does this qualify? I received the summons at about eight o'clock in the evening. Hjalmer, a logger, had not arrived home when it came on dark that frigid January night. His wife, Gert, went to the forty where he was working his contract.

Hearing the growl of his bulldozer, she stumbled toward it in the murk, picking her way through the debris of felled trees left by Hjalmer's efforts. The blade of the machine was lodged against the upright bole of a large tree, its treads chewing deep into frozen wood. Her husband was sprawled across the controls, crushed beneath a widow maker.

Loggers know all about widow makers. A dozer pushing against the trunk of a tree to tip it over instead jars its stronger base out from under its top, which then drops straight down onto the driver, onto Hjalmer. I have heard of this kind of thing happening when a heavy machine merely drives near the tree, its vibrations proving fatal.

I arrived at the scene, forty-five miles from town. Hjalmer had obviously been dead for hours. The ambient temperature was forty below zero, and he was frozen absolutely solid. Since it would be some time before anyone else could arrive, his wife helped me lever his body into the trunk of my car. In that unbendable state, his feet stuck out of the trunk. I prayed that darkness and snow swirled by my passage would obscure the fact.

When I patted Gert on the shoulder, she sniffled once and said, "Thanks, Doc. Drive careful, now."

. . .

Finding a remote country home from telephoned directions could be a test of concentration, requiring a knowledge of local history and a talent for extrapolation. "Go to Hank Cronson's old farm, turn left half a mile, take County 49. It ain't marked, Doc. Kids shot the sign all to hell. Turn sharp right. . . ." And so on.

Like this call: "We're the third house past the end of the

tarred part the road, Doc. Mailbox ain't got our name, been meanin' to paint something on it."

The problem? The road wore a tightly frozen veneer of compacted snow, which I had to stop and chisel off at regular intervals to see if the blasted pavement had quit.

. . .

Here's a house call of a different sort. Andy G. was a logging contractor who lived near Northpine. Each winter he and his wife moved to a shanty town of movable shacks housing his men near the job site, typically a place miles into the woods. Nearly every time I happened to bump into Andy in Northpine, he would insist that Barbara and I should stop by "the job" for a cup of coffee.

One night deputy sheriff Dick Ellison called just as Barbara and I were getting ready for bed. "Body found, Doc," he said apologetically. "Need the coroner. [Just one of the hats I wore at the time.] Want me to pick you up in my rig?" Barbara agreed to come along and act as recorder.

A young man's body lay trapped under his car at a spot some fifty-five miles from Northpine. After a couple stygian hours of crawling about in the muck, the sheriff decided that the victim, having parked his car on a slope, had had trouble starting it and had gone to the front of the vehicle and raised its hood, then had the misfortune to dislodge the car, which had rolled over him. He had not been found immediately.

Papers in the man's pocket suggested that he worked for Mr. Andy G. We sent the body back toward town in an ambulance, then drove some fifty miles in another black and wooded direction, hoping to discover Andy's camp.

The time was now about 3:00 AM. I knocked on the door of

a dark and quiet woodsman's shack. A spectral voice came from within. "Who's there?"

"Andy?" I called. "Doc MacDonald. You said for us to stop in for coffee sometime, so here we are."

I listened as the twang of social propriety stretched to its tensile limits and then heard, "One minute, Doc...."

Vivian

I FIRST MET VIVIAN about the time I began my practice. She lived more outdoors than in. Her delicately crinkled skin had been weathered by sixty-plus years of exposure to the northern climate, the effect akin to un-ironed fabric. Her complexion was a subdued bronze, courtesy of a dash of genes from Norway and a wealth from the Minnesota Ojibwe. She stood straight, her lean frame muscled from sawing and splitting firewood. Uncompromisingly gray hair was cut short enough not to be a bother. She lived alone in a cabin, a sixteen-by-twenty block of space enclosed by rustic walls that made it more an element of nature than an artifact of man. A clean interior testified to elbow grease and soap.

She had tried marriage and had borne a couple of children, since grown and off to lead lives in the city. She confided to me early on that she had tired of her husband's dedication to beer. He had returned one day, after the latest in a series of blackout drinking bouts, filled with the repentance a royal hangover inspires. She marched him through the doorway, then fished him out of a rill flowing past her house when he tumbled down its bank. Wet and bedraggled, he had trudged along the trail away from the cabin, disappearing from her life.

Vivian's cabin rested on land now claimed by the U.S. Forest Service. Right there, Indian values collided with Euro-American customs. To original Ojibwes, land had soul and was not something a human could own, any more than air to breathe or sun to warm. Officials from *Mikaduc Gov'ment*—Big Government—took comfort in fancies like deeds and titles and survey lines. An *Anishinaabeg*, a Person, subsisted frugally and gratefully on nature's gifts, his or her needs determining usage and "ownership."

A clerk in the regional forestry office noticed that Vivian had ignored a writ of—something or other—to vacate. Deputy sheriff Ike Strongbody was dispatched one sultry summer day to evict her. It happened that Ike bore about the same proportion of Scandinavian and Indian assets as did Vivian. He carried out the order of eviction by tacking it on the backside of a large pine tree where the only eyes to see it belonged to rabbits and the occasional wandering moose. The clerk was promoted to the city, and everyone in Northpine pretty much forgot about easing Vivian out of her home.

One day she sent word with trapper Jack Darnell that she would be pleased if I would stop by for a medical consultation. At the beginning of a practice, a young squirt of a doctor has plenty of blank lines on his appointment schedule. The day was one of those gorgeous October creations the north country does so well: maples red, aspens yellow, sturdy pines and spruce trees their steadfast green. A drive into the forest seemed a welcome substitute for sitting at a desk pretending to be busy.

To get to Vivian's place, I followed the U.S. highway for fifteen or sixteen miles, turned off on County 63, went on past George Johnson's old farm until a dirt track took off headed toward Canada, followed it to its second fork (the first being merely some road builder's miscalculation), and continued along the left branch for what was probably a mile. Maybe two. The trail tunneled beneath trees aflame with color, their leaves oddly luminescent in collaboration with a benign sun: a rainbow viewed from within.

Vivian was pulling carrots out of her garden when I arrived. She brushed loam from callused hands and clasped mine in her woodcutter's grip. We went into the cabin, where she offered me tea. North country etiquette dictates that one never refuse such a courtesy. Vivian took a handful of chopped tea leaves, tossed them in an old coffee can, and poured in steamy water. I had never before drunk tea so stout that the bottom of the cup hid from view even during the last quarter-inch. At length protocol was satisfied, and Vivian explained the reason for her summons, some medical problem. Details have escaped my memory because of what happened next.

I had grown up with only the skimpiest and most misinformed idea of Indian culture and temperament. A year of marriage to my Swedish/Ojibwe bride had shined a modest light onto Native society, and I had acquired that smidgen of knowledge which can still leave one short of true understanding.

Vivian left the door to her shack open while we discoursed. We sat facing each other, I turned away from the autumnal ostentation. She was just beginning to describe the medical issue I've forgotten when she rumbled, "Don't move, Doc. Don't even twitch."

I'm sure my hair would have stood on end had my style in those days not already been a butch. Vivian reached behind her and came out with a .410 shotgun.

"Steady, Doc."

Steady seemed a grand idea. I've tried to recall since if I remembered to breathe.

She raised the weapon.

Cowboy shows and James Fenimore Cooper tales rioted

through my brain. Dive for the floor? Grab the gun? Then I realized its barrel angled past my shoulder, and wild imaginings of ritual sacrifice gave way to a certainty that bears or pumas or tigers lurked. Well, maybe not tigers.

Vivian stood slowly and hissed, "Sit still." Then . . .

Do you know how loud a shotgun is when it goes off inside a shanty?

"Gotcha," Vivian crowed. I half expected her to blow smoke off the muzzle of that blunderbuss. She leaned her gun in the corner again.

"Pardon me, Doc." She strode out into the glorious sunshine and returned with a ruffed grouse dangling from one hand.

"Supper," she said. "Couldn't take a chance on him gettin' away."

Where There's the Will

Mrs. Ellen Sigworth sat on the edge of an examination table in Room Two of my office. Hard work's spoor roughened her hands and weathered her face, and a sheet covered her legs and lap. I dragged a chair to face her.

"What brings you today?" I chirped.

"I'm a little worried," she said.

I glanced at her chart. Married: yes, to Sam. Age: forty-seven. Vital signs recorded by nurse Verna Empey appeared benign. "What has you worried?" I asked.

"My monthlies are messed up."

"How so?"

"I spot a little nearly every day."

"Any cramps?"

"No, more of an ache down here." She flicked a hand across her lower abdomen.

"Hot flashes?" Incipient menopause?

"Only a few."

"Is there any chance that you might be pregnant?"

She grinned. "We'd better both hope not, Doc. Remember? You tied off Sam's what-cha-ma-call-its."

Ah yes, vasectomy. "Let's have a look."

Ellen's office call ceased to be routine the moment I inserted an examination speculum and saw her uterine cervix, the mouth of her womb. Angry, red, hard nodules of tissue obliterated normal anatomy. Palpation revealed that malignancy had swallowed her uterus and its neighboring tissues.

I needed no biopsy to know that Ellen had inoperable cancer of the uterine cervix. She faced scalding x-ray therapy and grinding agony during the few months she had left to live.

. . .

People of the far north are accustomed to isolation. The rules of survival: Make Do. Improvise. If established customs do not meet need, try something different.

In the late 1920s, Dr. George Papanicolaou first noticed that swabbings from a woman's uterine cervix could reveal the presence of cellular abnormalities that foretold the development of a lethal disease, cervical cancer. The famous Pap test was formally introduced to the profession in 1941, with the promise that if a woman destined to develop the malignancy had this simple test done annually, cancer of the cervix would disappear from mortality charts. Obviously, programs to provide this service in an affordable and convenient way would be standard by 1964.

Not so fast.

In my practice, I still found a victim of inoperable cervical cancer every year or two. Yet, like a good country doc, I did approximately two hundred Pap smears annually. It was easy to shrug and assign the deaths of those less foresighted to kismet. I'm doing my part. Can I help it if the *other* women don't come in for testing?

"Never heard of the test," Jane Doe says.

Madam, it's in all the newspapers. (Isn't it?) And I would have been glad to tell you about it, but you didn't—Ah, the cost. And the challenge of prying loose an appointment with the busy country doctor.

. . .

I moved my Minnesota practice from Littlefork to Grand Marais in April 1962. During the fall of 1964, an ad hoc group of service-minded people met to discuss forming a chapter of the American Cancer Society.

I have forgotten whose idea planted this seed. County nurse Ann Eliasen was present, and I was the designated doctor-type, rather reluctantly, I recall with chagrin. (It wasn't as though I, with my solo practice, lacked opportunities to keep busy.) I listened to my earnest compatriots working through the process of organizing, sidestepped the role of president, chairman, whatever. Kept track of the time. I'm not sure what caught my attention, but I suddenly realized these folks were sincere.

Someone asked me what a chapter of the American Cancer Society should do.

"Be opposed to cancer," I suggested.

I got *looks* from the rest of them.

"Maybe—do something about cancer."

"What, Doctor?"

What? "Well, tell people the signs to look for?"

"I think that's in newspapers already," one of the ladies muttered.

Do something!

Show an informational movie? Well, I'd tried that the year before. The Lions Club, looking for a program, asked me to present a medical topic. Now I, a non-smoker, had grown hoarse from bad-mouthing the use of tobacco. Skeptical Puffer Patient Number 3915 says, "I've been smoking for seventy-five years and it hasn't hurt me one bit. [Cough, strangle, cough.] 'Sides, I can quit any time I want to."

Time for an object lesson, good Lions? I selected a film on lung cancer, scheduled for right after lunch. Are all you sated Lions comfy? An X-rated movie, this, complete with scenes from the operating room and pathology lab. Whoops! Two Lions on the floor, the lavatory clogged.

Dear reader, do you relish graphic views of what is happening "under the hood" of a human body? No? Perhaps my Lions were not unique. So, what would be Cancer Society-ish without endangering the composure of our audience?

"Wellll," I hedged, thinking: do something, say something, act as though you know where we are headed.

I remembered Dr. Papanicolaou and his marvelous test. "Maybe we could sponsor clinics, provide free or low-cost screening sessions."

The ladies leaped on the idea like a duck on a June bug. I realized I had just made another commitment to busyness.

Seeking sponsorship, we approached the American Cancer Society with our plan. The response: Not interested. Forget it. Sorry. Nada. We'll call you. Sayonara.

"But we just want you to—"

"No funds for that kind of thing! Count us out."

"We aren't asking for money. We just thought it fit the mission of your organization."

No response.

We wrote again. "Could you, would you endorse our efforts, gratis?"

A letter came in reply. "What?"

We used simple language: "No money. Use your name."

"Really? Well . . . okay."

The following spring, we scheduled a series of "Pap clinics," one each weekend during April, to coincide with the society's Cancer Awareness Month. All participating professionals—physicians, nurses, lab technicians, other helpers—would donate their time and talents. We prayed that a few ladies would show up.

Three hundred fifty women came to that first round of clinics. Dr. Wallace Smith, a thirty-year veteran of medical practice in Grand Marais, a wonderful, unassuming, insightful physician who became one of my closest friends, and I did all of the pelvic examinations, collecting the Pap smears. Dr. Arthur Wells, pathologist at St. Luke's Hospital in Duluth, examined the samples for a fee of three dollars each—below the going rate, and the total cost to the ladies who participated.

That first year we found four positive smears, each representing an early—curable—stage of cancer. In a small community like ours, news of this magnitude spreads from grateful patient to distant cousin before nightfall.

For the next twenty-six years, April was the community's cancer-screening month. The American Cancer Society decided that what we had accomplished warranted more than a letter. They regularly sent representatives to monitor the process, and awards and placards from the national office arrived each spring, bundled up with the seed catalogues.

A cadre of women, credited in this book's appendix, coalesced around the original group of helpers. Newly appointed county public health nurse Rosemary Lamson took over from Ann Eliasen when she retired. After the first couple of years, Dr. Wells used his persuasive skills on his Duluth colleagues, and seven or eight city specialists joined us so that we could add breast examinations to the routine.

Attending one of the cancer clinics required an investment of three to four hours of a woman's time. Fees were never more than the actual cost of supplies and reading the slides. Under the prods of inflation and the expanding number of tests available, the fee gradually rose to a maximum of eighteen dollars. To keep those who were waiting busy, Ms. Lamson added to the scope of the visit, offering half-a-dozen assessments for non-cancerous problems, including blood pressure checks, blood tests for cholesterol and sugar, and urinalyses and stool tests for hidden blood. During peak years, between five and six hundred women came through the clinics annually, this out of a total county population of just over four thousand citizens, male and female, young and old. Judging from the buzz in the waiting area outside our examination rooms, I concluded that the ladies were having a ball. Sisters in misery? After all, who really wants to go through *that* kind of exam? Still, it sounded as though they were having fun. Self-help of a unique type: I'm convinced that's why the idea worked.

A few colleagues scoffed at the thought of dispensing free care. Yet I found that the number of Pap smears I did in the office remained steady at about two hundred each year. Ninety-nine percent of participants came from our own "catchment area"; less than a handful were "outsiders." I concluded that the bulk of these patients would not otherwise have had the test done at all.

It was a rare year in which we did not turn up at least one positive test. In addition, other tumors—of the breast, ovaries, or skin—were discovered. Were the clinics worth the effort? Perhaps those whose lives were rescued might be best qualified to answer.

Along about the tenth or twelfth year, a contingent of guys approached county nurse Lamson, a distinct chip on their collective shoulders. They wanted a cancer screening session for men.

Doctors Warren Brooker (intern-mate and lifelong friend) and Mac Fifield, urologists in Duluth, promptly agreed to join forces with us. We offered free screening clinics for cancer of the prostate and other genital organs. In the first year, we found four cases of prostate cancer, plus one of testicular cancer.

The gist of this is simple: if we doctors are serious about making effective screening tests readily available to the general public, then we need to do *our* part to make them readily available to the general public. Elementary, my dear Watson. During the twenty-seven consecutive years that the Cook County Cancer Screening Clinics were held, 12,111 examinations were performed on women attendees, an average enrollment of 450. Beginning in 1974 and continuing for eighteen years, the men's version of the cancer clinic saw 4,951 examinations performed, a yearly average of 275.

As for the "economics"—a dastardly word when it intrudes into matters of health—I found that I lost little if any income. In fact, we often discovered conditions that I would then be consulted for in my office: an unsuspected diabetic, or someone with albumen in the urine or occult blood in a stool sample.

This approach to preventive medicine was unorthodox, almost serendipitous. Turn loose a group of ambitious, motivated volunteers on a self-help project and marvelous things can occur.

Where there's the will—

Maud and Lars

WHEN I ARRIVED IN NORTHPINE in January 1948, the logging business was nearing the end of an era. Woods workers were giants in the land, though not necessarily in stature. Many of the old "jacks" I got to know, to admire, were wiry men, even scrawny, but they were durable as rawhide left in rain and sun and wind.

Until about 1940, a contractor would typically establish a camp near where logs were to be harvested. Roads were scarce across the northern reaches of Minnesota. Even those present were at the mercy of season and weather, often quagmires of primal mud unless frozen solid by winter's uncompromising decree. Rivers provided the means of transport. The last recorded drive, a flotilla of humping, grinding logs pouring downstream in a northern river swollen by melted snow, occurred in 1935 on the Little Fork River. Flickering images of the event exist on black-and-white movie film in an historical interpretive center located outside of Grand Rapids, Minnesota.

Maud was a head cook, a refugee from the days when camps were the rule. Camp cooks were jewels to be treated with special respect. The head cook was the boss, and the bull cook, or assistant, was typically a bruiser who could ride herd on "da boys" if they got out of hand. There was no lumberjack Maud could not stare down or arm wrestle into submission, if necessary. A large woman, buxom—a blacksmith in skirts.

Maud was content with her life in the woods. Then, progress in its insidious fashion waylaid the logging business, and the camps began to close. All Maud knew was how to cook for "da boys," and, with no ready alternative in sight, she awoke one day to the realization that she needed another venue in life. Among "da boys" at Maud's table one winter near the end of the thirties was a mild, quiet man named Lars, the last jack in camp to start trouble. Maud looked the field over and decided on Lars.

"Da boys" tended to head for Northpine or International Falls after the camps closed for summer's wet season. With pockets full of winter's earnings, they were ready for a soiree. Lars had no other thought in mind, but there were Maud and her plans. She and Lars honeymooned while the rest of "da boys" were whooping it up in Chisholm and Duluth.

Life flowed on after this unexpected jog in its even course. Maud and Lars had themselves three kids, all girls. She cooked for Lars, but, truth to tell, it was hard cutting recipes to one-table size. Through it all, Lars remained calm, laconic, and as skinny as he had been during his logging days. With only one husband and three kids to manage, Maud gave them a full camp's worth of bossing. Mostly Lars would smile in his quiet, almost, well, *sweet* way, paying as little attention to all the instructions as he could arrange. Internal earflaps work so much better than the kind that fasten on the outside.

Now, jump ahead three decades, for that's when Lars and Maud became my patients.

Lars began to lose weight. Since there was little fat on his frame to begin with, it didn't take long for this state of affairs to show. Maud herded him into the office that first time.

I asked Lars my usual opening gambit, "What brings you here today?"

Maud said, "He don't eat."

Weight loss, anorexia: could mean trouble in a sixty-five-year-old. "Do you have any pain?" I asked.

"He don't have any pain; he just won't eat."

I explained to Maud that I wanted to get information straight from the source. She favored me with the look that had straightened out many a mess-hall ruckus.

I asked my questions with only a modicum of help from Maud. Or from Lars, for that matter, that taciturn business. I ordered the battery of tests and internal investigations such symptoms demand.

We reconvened ten days later. There were no positive findings to discuss, but three fewer pounds on Lars increased my concerns. I explained the results—rather, the lack thereof—and confessed that I had no explanation for his continuing weight loss.

"He don't eat," Maud muttered.

"I've decided that he should be seen by an internal medicine specialist down on the Iron Range," I explained. Lars smiled his quiet little smirk; Maud fluttered her hands, muttering.

Dr.—I'll call him Dr. X.—sent me a letter after re-exploring Lars's innards and blood. His findings coincided with mine: no obvious explanation for Lars's mysterious weight loss. Although Dr. X. thanked me for sending this "interesting case," I carried away his unwritten hope that I would refrain from any similar referrals in the future.

A week later I received a frantic call from Maud at her home.

Lars had weakened to the point that he had fallen and could not get up off the floor. Before I could knock, Maud jerked open the door to their modest bungalow and yanked me across the threshold. Lars, skeletal, lay on his back, hands folded across his skinny abdomen. He smiled at me placidly.

Maud charged back and forth from the kitchen to the living room, where I knelt beside Lars. She thrust a plate of fried chicken under my nose.

"See? He wouldn't eat it! Says it gives him the pukes! What am I to do? Make him eat, Doctor!"

Cutting through the bee-hum drone of Maud's lament, I tried to question Lars and finally called for the ambulance. At the hospital I ordered intravenous fluids and high-calorie supplements. Lars pulled out the IV needles, refused any nutritional rocket boosters, would not allow me to put a feeding tube into his stomach. I was by now as worried as Maud.

I sent Lars to a psychiatrist on the Iron Range. His report had overtones similar to that of Dr. X. Since Lars was an adult, and since he was not really incompetent—"a little crazy, but not in any legal sense"—the psychiatrist had no suggestions. He shipped Lars back to the Northpine Hospital.

I rounded up Lars's daughter Martha, the only one of his children locally available. I explained that her father was actually going to die if he did not abandon his hunger strike. Martha dabbed at her cheeks and said, "I grew up with those two. Mom telling everyone when to breathe and how deep; Pa smiling but paying no attention."

I collected Maud and Martha, and we confronted Lars in his bed.

"Lars, I find it intolerable that you will not let us help you. Is there something—anything—you want to tell us? Please?"

Maud muttered, "He just won't *eat!*"

Lars smiled in his sweet way and looked out the window.

He died five days later.

I could not put the actual cause of death on that form the State of Minnesota expects me to fill out. Instead I called it inanition, a gold-plated word for starvation. What I dared not record was:

Lars had found a way to get even with Maud.

My Very Last Home Delivery

HAVING BABIES is a natural process, condoned by nature over the eons. Midwives have plied their craft from times retreating through a misty past to the origin of our species. Obstetricians—doctors to assist the process—are a far more recent idea. When it comes to birthing babies, the newest wrinkle of all is the idea of doing so in a hospital.

During the early years of my practice, I offered patients the option of a home delivery. A few took me up on it, often, we discovered, when poverty made a hospital stay an impossible expense. A delivery-room nurse by special training, Barbara accompanied me when summoned to some backwoods cabin.

January and February were the coldest months in Northpine country. One thirty-below night Barbara and I were snuggled in our bed when the telephone rang. I groped for the receiver.

"Hello?"

A woman's voice said, "Doc MacDonald? Listen, Babe's in labor and it ain't comin' right. We-uns need you right lively."

"Babe who?"

"Well, her name's actual Josephine Meyers, but we-uns call her—Look, Doc she's screamin' her head off, how it hurts, and the kid won't come."

"Sounds as though you had better bring her in to the hospital."

"There isn't time, and, 'sides, we don't have a car what'll start and it's so cold out, dassn't bring her. We live on the old Horekoski farm, two miles west a Sarah Lake on County 49, then south five miles on 36, then west a quarter mile to a drive-way pullin' to the right. Got that? Hurry, Doc."

Click. Dial tone.

I jiggled the phone's shut-off lever. "Hello! Dang." Sarah Lake, I thought? It's thirty-five miles away on the U.S. high-way, then. . . . I turned on the bedside light and clutched at the shirttails of fleeing memory to scribble the woman's further instructions.

I poked Barbara's shoulder. "Wake up."

She twitched.

"Home delivery," I said.

She whispered, "Have fun."

I poked again. "You signed on to help, remember?"

"You believed me?" She pulled the covers over her head.

"Barb!"

"Oh, okay." She made a production out of pulling on her nurse's garb.

We carried an already-assembled pack on our home deliveries, sterilized and wrapped securely. We persuaded our battered Ford to creak into motion, its suspension system squeaking from the cold. When we reached the highway and headed south from Northpine, Barbara asked, "Who is our patient?"

"A woman named Meyers. Recall her?"

"We have no one on our list of pregnant patients named Meyers."

"I was afraid that might be the case."

"And where are we headed?"

"Sarah Lake and ... here, I wrote down the rest." I handed her my scrawled note.

She squinted. "You'll have to read that yourself, Doctor. I doubt the pharmacist could decipher this. Are you sure you weren't just dreaming?"

"No, no, I answered the phone." I did, didn't I? Good Lord, what if it *was* a dream?

Barbara glanced at me. "Let me see if I have this right. We're headed out on a frigid night to someplace you're not sure of, to deliver a woman we never heard of, maybe?"

"The woman said she.... Maybe I should have gotten more precise information."

Barbara crossed her arms in that way she had when I'd done something unusually boneheaded.

We found the Meyers homestead. The house was an ungainly, two-story clapboard building looming out of moonless darkness in an unlit farmyard. We collected supplies and groped along a narrow path wainscoted with four feet of snow. I pounded on a battered wood-paneled door, which opened on hinges complaining like the gate of a sepulcher. Light oozed from a kerosene lamp held aloft by a woman whose face made sixty look like a war lost. She grunted, "Took ya long enough. In here."

We followed her through a kitchen, into a second room containing a sofa with grotesquely lumpy cushions, a small dining table, a pair of cane-bottom chairs, a chest gap-toothed with one missing drawer, and that ubiquitous heater of the far north, a rumbling wood-burning barrel stove. A frowzy double bed stood in one corner.

Our guide set the lamp atop the chest. Glancing around,

I made out a woman's form on the bed. She lay tautly, a blanket clutched, wadded, in both hands. She peered at us like a spooked deer in the forest, atremble. I stood beside her and gently felt her swollen abdomen.

"You are?" I asked.

"Her-uns is Babe," the older woman said. "Told you that."

I glanced back at her. "And you are?"

"Her Ma, Dolly Quiggly."

I turned back to Babe. "Who is your regular doctor?"

Dolly said, "You are."

"But I've never seen her."

"She-uns been meanin' to come in; hadn't got around to it."

"Who were you planning to have deliver her?"

"I've done that a time or two."

"Any prenatal care?"

"What's that?"

"Is this her first baby?"

"Yep."

Great. "I'll need to check—"

Babe erupted. She arched her back and screamed in a voice roughened from hours of strain, writhing and tearing at the blanket. When the labor contraction ceased, the exhausted woman collapsed within herself, eyes closed, sweat dripping down grimy cheeks. "Open the delivery pack," I murmured to Barbara and pulled on a sterile glove to examine the woman. When I separated her legs, I first noticed that she had had polio during her youth. One leg was a wasted stick: skin, bone, virtually absent muscle.

Barbara crawled onto the bed and soothed Babe, holding her leg while I checked the position of the baby in the birth canal.

Oh, God.

The baby lay in what is termed a frank breech position. Its legs were swept up to lie beside the head and its buttocks were coming first.

A breech delivery is always more hazardous to the baby than the preferred head-first version. Add the facts that this was a first pregnancy, that this breech presentation was the most difficult type to deliver, that the woman's pelvis had been warped by polio, that the "delivery room" was in a home where poverty ruled, nearly sixty miles from our hospital, that after more than twenty-four hours of labor Babe was exhausted....

I believe every doctor has a secret "what the hell am I doing here?" button hidden away in his psyche. Some emergencies seem unsolvable. I will never forget those seconds during which I had to face the reality of Babe and her child: the patient's terror and pain; the total lack of sterile or usual working conditions; the stigmata of poverty, a clinging miasma; the absence of light; open-drop chloroform the only possible anesthetic because of the grumbling wood stove, a threat to ether's volatility; the numbing realization that I had no alternative but to solve the problem.

I concocted a delivery table of sorts: tip the two chairs back against the edge of the bed and swivel poor Babe so they could serve as leg supports; place Barbara on the bed to pour chloroform and to hold the desperate woman in place.

I said to Dolly, "Do you have a flashlight somewhere?"

She found one in the spavined chest of drawers.

"Good," I said. "Stand behind me and shine it onto Babe so that I can see what—"

A contraction began. Babe screamed and sobbed in total despair. The baby's buttocks showed at the opening of the birth canal. "Push," Barbara and I implored. Babe screamed anew and kicked me in the chest with her good leg. The chairs tumbled behind me. I groped deeply into the birth canal, Babe's leg now resting on my shoulder. The woman tore her vocal chords asunder.

It dawned on Dolly Quiggly that "things were not going well." She departed for the kitchen at a run, taking the flashlight with her. We could hear her shouting at God.

Babe's ability to feel pain was nearly bankrupt. I reached far into the logjam created by a baby chest, head, and legs, found a foot, commanded knee and hip joints to function, and finally dragged down one leg. Space gained. Found the second; slid it free. The baby moved down the birth canal, and I eased its head past the last grip of the womb and pelvis.

Baby girl Meyers lay limp in my hands. She made no effort to breathe. I squeezed her chest and released it with a snap. No response. I yanked down my face mask and covered the infant's face with my mouth.

Puff air into lungs fragile as soap bubbles.

Squeeze air out.

Repeat.

Set up a rhythm. Air in, squeeze out. Over and over.

She opened her eyes and raised tiny arms in a startle position. I puffed harder.

Was her skin turning pink?

She tried a breath of her own. A mew like that of a kitten just arrived.

I puffed again.

She screwed up her face in annoyance.

I snapped the bottoms of her feet, and she bent her knees to escape my finger.

A gasp. A cough. She drew breath deep enough to swear at

me in baby talk. She shut her eyes and began to cry with a will. Her skin turned rosy.

Papa Meyers appeared from upstairs, on a narrow stairway set into one corner.

"What is it?" he demanded.

"A girl," I said. "A gutsy, tough, wonderful little girl."

"A girl? Shit." Papa headed back upstairs.

We unraveled in reverse the maze connecting the Meyers home with Northpine, just as the sun peered over a frosty eastern horizon. Barbara cried softly into a sodden handkerchief. "What chance does she have?" she muttered.

"Our chief of obstetrics always said, 'Just deliver them; don't try to love them.'"

"You don't mean that!"

"Sure I do." I bruised a fist against the dashboard.

Esther

S O FAR AS I COULD TELL, Esther was a normal seven-pound lass when she was born early one morning in the Northpine Hospital. Her mother's labor had been uneventful, the delivery spontaneous, and I detected no abnormalities in Esther then or during the two or three days she was a guest in the hospital nursery. She was about a month old when I saw her next, for a routine postnatal checkup.

There was a horrendous systolic murmur across the front of Esther's chest.

How could an infant acquire such an obvious and ominous rumble in the short space of one month? Had I missed it during her stay in the hospital? The murmur shook the baby's chest wall and filled the ear pieces of my stethoscope with a growl mindful of a diesel motor.

Esther's heart had a large opening between its two pumping chambers, what doctors term an interventricular septal defect. Such a mistake of nature only makes a sound when there is a difference in liquid pressure between the two chambers (a state normally present inside an intact heart), allowing blood to flow in an abnormal direction. At birth and for a brief time after, the pressure differences have not developed; hence, no murmur initially. The defect, remedial at the time Esther was born, required open-heart surgery to close it. I contacted the department of cardiac surgery at the university and made arrangements for little Esther to be seen by experts at the medical center.

Emergencies are relative. Large institutions demand that reams of paperwork be prepared in advance of any procedures, and a month drifted by while official gears ground through orthodoxy. Then—

Esther's mother was as white as the infant was blue when they arrived in our emergency room. Esther bubbled, fighting for air, her body swollen with edema, backed-up fluid. She was in massive heart failure. Digitalis, originally extracted from the foxglove plant, was the profession's quick fix for a flailing heart, but I had never before been faced with "digitalizing" a patient so small. Dosage is based on weight, so after extrapolating from a usual dose, I injected the antidote, along with a diuretic to release fluid. It worked. A quick telephone call to my specialist colleagues at the university, and Esther was on her way to the Twin Cities, nearly three hundred miles away. She had her operation, the hole was closed, and her prognosis became good.

A particular pleasure for a country doctor is watching kids arrive and then monitoring them as they mature. Time did its thing, and Esther, now a teen, decided to participate in one of the high school athletic programs. She arrived at the office one day for a physical examination. A patient like Esther is always a delight to the doctor who was there when things were not going well. We chatted, I listened to her chest in a doctorly way, and—wait. Her pulse was slow: forty-four beats a minute. I have read that great runners have so developed their cardiovascular systems that they exhibit such nonchalant pulses, but Esther? I had her do thirty seconds' worth of jumping jacks and checked again: forty-four. A minute of exercise: forty-four.

"How are you feeling?" I asked.

"Okay." She drew a deep breath. "Maybe a little light-headed."

I ordered an EKG, an electrical tracing of heart activity. Esther was in complete heart block: something had interfered with the electrical impulses that tell the heart's pumping chambers when and how fast to beat. Nature's last-resort safety circuits were keeping her going. I sent Esther back to the university.

When an especially large opening in the heart must be sewn shut, an ever-present danger is that a stitch or subsequent scarring from the operation will pinch off the "wires" carrying messages to the pumping chambers. This had obviously happened to Esther. The solution: a lifelong indwelling pacemaker. Esther has worn one for years now, and her life is normal. I often cast memory back to the day that blue, puffy little girl arrived in our emergency room. I offer thanks that she lives in the medical times that she does.

Assumptions

PROBLEM: doctors, as mere human beings, can never park humanity on some shelf when consulted by a patient. Essential when an empathetic ear is required, this very humanity also leads a doctor into leaps of conjecture as surely as it does Mr. Jones down the block. Frantic telephone calls prophesying doom stir those adrenal glands and "Oh, no!" brain centers of the physician right along with those of the caller.

Accidents provide many of the unscheduled patients a country doctor sees. A fishhook in the body tourist, a skier twisting a leg bone beyond its torsional strength, a tree or pile of logs landing on human parts less sturdy than they. And is there a more deadly profession than that of farming?

A regular source of "business" in my practice was the U.S. highway passing through Northpine, connecting Canada with more settled parts of Minnesota. At certain times of year the highway sees caravans of travelers.

One day I received a phone call from our sheriff. He sounded worried. "A tanker hauling diesel rolled over, the driver inside. On fire. Hurry, Doc."

I set out, dread a familiar dragon gnawing at my gut. For an isolated rural physician, there is an ever-looming self-doubt regarding competency for the task thrust upon him.

The wreck was six miles south of town. I drove toward a huge pillar of greasy black smoke, a further goad to anxiety, and approached the usual knots of cars clustered on either side of the blazing truck. I bulled my way through, got clearance from highway patrolman Curt Innes when he recognized me, and parked a couple hundred feet away, wondering, does diesel fuel ever explode?

I joined Curt and deputy sheriff Tom Ejerdahl, standing as close as heat would allow. "Fire truck en route," Tom said. "It's burning like the produce truck that crashed in the middle of the night that time, its two drivers incinerated. Leaves a man helpless. Ah, here come the firemen."

The truck cab and its attached tanker-trailer lay on their sides in a ditch beside the road. I watched while my neighbors and friends on the volunteer fire department edged close, doing their jobs for the simple reason they needed doing. I waited while they squirted and foamed, and I tried to peer into the inferno that was the cab and its contents. No body visible, no blackened skulls engulfed in dirty flame, as there had been in the other tragedy. How long could human flesh withstand such heat? Once Death confirmed its visit, I would switch hats from physician to county coroner.

I joined a circle of gawkers around an industrial-age bonfire. One of the firemen duck-walked close enough to peer through the gap where the windshield had been. He crawled away and slogged toward Sheriff Ejerdahl.

"I can't see anything that looks like human remains," he reported. "Unless the body burned completely."

A burly fellow standing a few feet away heard and approached. "You looking for the driver? That's me. I clumb out through the front window of the cab just as she went up."

. . .

The usual quota of summertime patients jammed my office anteroom, those awaiting past-due appointments crammed next to unscheduled walk-ins and tourists. Receptionist Lila grabbed my coattails to announce that someone from the local Coast Guard station had called: one of their number had fallen from the top of a thirty-foot flagpole and would be arriving momentarily. I groaned, silently, I think. A disaster on top of an increasingly surly contingent already waiting? I had learned the best preparation for some vague pending calamity: plod along, do what I could to clear the decks. I plodded.

A half hour went by without the banshee wail of a siren or a summons to the hospital emergency room. Good Lord, could it possibly be a coroner case by now? I worked on, wondering. An hour elapsed. By then I had become entangled in the tribulations of those streaming through the office and nearly forgot about the looming disaster.

I took the spanking new chart of one Arthur DCamp and eased into Room Three. Age: twenty-two. A sturdy lad, speckled—I adjusted my glasses—with freckles of white paint?

"Mr. DCamp," I said, "what brings you here today?"

"They insisted."

"For starters, who is 'they'?"

"Well, actually, the chief."

Now we're getting somewhere. "Who is the chief?"

"Fella named John Johnson."

Solid data. Still—Try another tack. "You say Chief Johnson insisted. How do *you* feel about—" I winced at the insidious afterglow of a recent symposium on office-practice counseling. Sighing, I glanced at my watch. "What's wrong?"

"Not really all that much." He held up a sturdy pinky.

Ye gods, has a new code been assigned to another of the upper-extremity digits?

Arthur grinned, rather sheepishly, I thought.

"Tell me what happened that made the chief demand you come here and—" And wave a little finger at me.

"Well, see, Doc, like, I'm doing maintenance around the Coast Guard base, and the chief decides the flagpole could use a coat of paint, and, see, I'm not what you call a steeplejack, and, see, I climb up that stupid thing and get my bucket of paint all ready when, *whoosh,* the dang belt sorta lets loose, and down I come, *kerplunk,* until it fetches up on a crossbar nailed to the pole at about four feet off the ground. Doc, see, my feet hits the ground at the same instant, and I sorta lose my balance, like, and tip over backwards, ass pointin' toward the sun, and land dab on my little finger. I think it's, like, sprained."

See, he was, like, right on.

Bill Makos

M Y FATHER-IN-LAW was a massive man, a gentle man, a respected elder of Minnesota's Chippewa Tribe. Shortly after I married his daughter, he asked if I would consider providing remote Chippewa Lake Reservation with some kind of medical service. I explained all the reasons why it was impractical: distance, time away from Northpine, lack of acceptable facilities on site. In short, I said yes.

That's how it happened that for several years I traveled to the reservation once a week to hold a "clinic." Chippewa Lake, the body of water, was a remote pond some four or five miles across, wild rice growing in profusion along its shores. In 1949, wild rice was still *wild* rice: *mahnomen.* Providing a traditional food source for the woodland Indians living in the area, as it had for centuries before we Caucasians arrived, its sale was one of the few sources of cash available to the people living there. Gathering it from a canoe, roasting it to drive off moisture, trampling it with moccasined feet to separate seed from hull, winnowing it—the process came as close to preservation of tradition as anything history had bequeathed the Chippewa Lakers.

Every Tuesday noon my wife, Barbara, an RN, and I loaded our old Ford with medical supplies and headed south along State Highway 65 toward Chippewa Lake, some fifty-five miles away. In those days, the road was a lane-and-a-half-wide track, rutted, sandy or muddy, winding past swamps, rivers of somber brown water, trees in glorious profusion, and prodigious rocks deposited by some absent-minded glacier.

At that time, about five hundred people lived scattered on the sprawling reservation, an area of twelve hundred square miles. Perhaps half of the people lived in a compact village on the eastern shore of the lake. Our "office" was a nook in the village's old boxy wooden elementary school. Despite the Spartan facilities, I really liked that office. Good things happened in its dingy confines.

One afternoon as Barbara and I stowed away supplies after another busy clinic, silver-haired Old Bill Makos appeared at the top of the stairway.

"Doc, my Mary and I were wondering if you and Barbara would care to have supper with us before you head home."

Barbara spoke for us. "We'd love to. You can tell me more stories about my dad from back in the old days."

Bill said, grinning, "I've got something to show you, and a small favor to ask."

We trotted after him, trying to keep up with his brisk gait. His home stood just across the road from the schoolhouse. He paused before the door of his garage, posed like a magician about to amaze and astound, and opened it with a flourish.

On the garage floor were five fish. *Huge* fish. I learned that they ranged in size from thirty-five to eighty-seven pounds.

"What *are* they?" I asked.

Bill smiled full bore, his eyelids nearly closed. "Sturgeon. They come up the stream leading out of Chippewa Lake to spawn. My son Ira, Fatty Woodstock, and I catch them." He squinted in glee again. "Care to guess how we do that? No hooks, no nets."

"Uh, dynamite?"

"Bah! Tomfoolery. We use traditional methods." He produced a pole twelve or fourteen feet long, a hank of clothesline threaded through a series of screw eyelets fastened along its length.

I said, "Traditional? I dunno, Bill. That looks a lot like whiteman, hardware-store stuff."

He waggled a finger at me. "Picky, picky, Doc. One of us stands on a rock in the river, near a shallow rapids; someone else on shore hangs onto the free end of rope. When the fish swims up the rapids, the top of its tail fin sticks out of the water. You just slip a loop of rope around its tail and snug it up. Then's when the fun begins. Eighty pounds of sturgeon puts up a fuss!" He nudged a water pail with his foot. "This here is fish eggs. Caviar. Old Doc Hanover is always after me to send him some. Thought maybe you could take it back to him."

I grinned delightedly. *Old* Doc Hanover? It wasn't often I got one up on my mentor, middle-aged Dr. Ralph.

Bill said, "We're having sturgeon for supper."

I thought, I hope they taste better than they look. Rarely indeed have looks been so deceiving.

After supper, Bill, Mary, Barbara, and I sat in the Makos living room.

"What has it been like for you, your visits down here?" Bill asked.

"Fascinating. People I'd never have met otherwise. A sense that what we're doing is useful. I've learned firsthand what it feels like to stand out because of appearance; here I'm the minority. But it's frustrating: so many health problems."

"We've never had on-site medical care before, us fifty-five

miles from anywhere. Trouble piles up. Tell me, honestly, what do you see as the biggest concern?"

"Well—you asked, Bill—I'd say the big three at the clinic, in terms of frequency, are impetigo, terribly bad teeth, and chronically infected, running ears, with hearing a casualty in those cases."

"Others?"

"Endless respiratory infections. Diarrheas. Poor nutrition. Inadequate prenatal care. Lack of immunizations—there Barbara and I have had some impact. Scabies. Lice. I suppose poverty and dismal housing are behind some of that."

"But they don't have to be," Bill said softly. "You didn't mention alcohol."

"I know it's a problem, but in the year we've been coming now, I haven't had a single inebriated patient in the office."

"These people respect you two," Bill said softly.

My eyes misted. "Bill, you obviously have had education. Where?"

"Carlyle Indian School in Pennsylvania."

"Isn't that where Jim Thorpe attended?"

"I played football with him." He grinned. "Mostly I tried to stay out of his way, the same as I would a Peterbilt truck. I lived outside the reservation for a while. It was . . . all right. Then I came back here. It was . . . easier. A man has to live somewhere. Here, among my people, I'm judged by the kind of person I am. Out there. . . ." He shrugged.

"Ah," I said, glancing at Barbara. "Prejudice."

Bill studied me, and I felt a flash of tension. What was he expecting? "Your look is saying something."

He sighed. "What is your heritage?"

"Besides American? Celtic. Scottish. A generous dash of Irish."

"And your profession?"

I cocked an eyebrow. "Why, medicine."

He squinted. "Medicine. You didn't say it was 'being Scottish.'"

"I seldom think about—Oh."

His smile was pensive. "Whenever someone meets you, they likely say and think, 'Hello, Doctor.' Not, 'Hello, Scotsman.' When someone new sees me, my role is, first of all, being Indian. You can be 'a doctor who also happens to be'—like that—while my brothers and I, wherever we go, are 'an Indian who is—what?' But Indian first! My character or abilities are always afterthoughts, if they come up at all."

We talked long. Bill invited me to attend a powwow, a real one, with a nighttime wood fire, the thump and wail that span the centuries, garb that was no longer a "costume." I thrill to the music of Bach and Brahms and Beethoven. A dance done by *Anishinaabeg*, the People, for the people is a spiritual event. For me, that music rates with the masters.

I cherish your legacy, Bill (Little Bear) Makos.

The Human Essence

A HIGHLIGHT OF MY PROFESSIONAL CAREER was an opportunity to teach at the University of Minnesota Medical School in Minneapolis. A program designed in 1970 by Dr. John Verby, MD, called the Rural Physician Associate Program, or, more affectionately, R-PAP, placed third-year medical students in the offices of selected small-city and rural practitioners. Goals of R-PAP included the hope that city-bred students could be shown the advantages and satisfactions of a rural life. Not only did this strategy work, the experience turned out to be an all-around educational gem as well.

My involvement with the program allowed me to travel Minnesota from border to border, spending entire days in one-on-one contact with the individual students. I supervised patient encounters and videotaped, for student review, half-a-dozen in-depth patient interviews over the course of a year at each location. "In-depth" meant delving into the person's psycho/social/sexual life as well as obtaining essential biological information.

Busy physicians cut corners. I was as guilty of "hurry-up" medical interviews as any of my harassed colleagues. The issues that emerged under the mandated but gentle, often timid, and persistent questioning by the student regularly left student, me, and the patient's personal physician agape at what we had learned.

. . .

Automat Medicine—quickie diagnosis and even quicker therapy via prescription pad—carries with it the certainty that many a patient's real needs are not discovered. Psychiatrist Carl Jung wrote, "Man is something more than intellect, emotion, and two dollar's worth of chemicals," postulating the need for what has come to be called "spirituality." When does the concept belong in the office of a busy physician? Hilda comes to mind.

Myron was my R-PAP student for the day, and Hilda, a solemn, subdued, middle-aged woman, rotund and matronly, was his interviewee. A good student, Myron sailed through the essential medical information and did a fine job of eliciting the psycho/social/sexual information most of us doctors find difficult to ask about. Then he asked if she had ever been abused.

It was as if Myron had turned some switch. Hilda sat erect, and the nearly disinterested look on her face vanished. She smiled, a Mona Lisa grimace. "What do you consider abuse?" she asked.

Myron said, "Well . . . why don't you tell me?"

"I belonged to—" she mentioned a Christian church with a reputation for fundamentalist beliefs. She stared over Myron's shoulder, and some deep reverie descended upon her.

"I was sixteen," she said softly. "Brother Pangborn was our minister. It was during Sunday morning service." She found a handkerchief. "That was more than twenty years ago. I still waken some nights with his voice roaring in my ears, his face looming over me.

"He called me to the altar that day, made me stand beside him, in front of the congregation. 'Brothers! Sisters!' Brother Pangborn shouted. 'Hilda has a *special* testimony to give.' There, before my parents, before my friends, all those gaping people, he made me confess that I had been with ... that my boyfriend and I ... that I was pregnant. I tried to get him to quit, stammered, 'I ... sinned....' Brother Pangborn was sweating when he glared down at me.

"I said, 'We ... we love each other,' but he just screamed, 'Sinner!' I remember being so puzzled. How can love be a bad thing? He kept yelling at me, 'Do you repent?' Finally I just yelled back at him, 'No! In the name of Christ, leave me alone!'

"I fled down the aisle," still-suffering, middle-aged Hilda said softly, "and I've never set foot in that place again, but that day my parents stayed until the service ended."

Hilda sobbed into her hands, then mopped with her hankie. "I had decided that since I was such a rotten person, I would go home and—and kill myself. Then I remembered about baby and realized I couldn't choose for her. She's twenty-three now, out of college, and—Doctor, she's a *fine* woman."

Myron leaned forward and took her hand in both of his. I saw tears on his cheeks. He said, "What have you decided about yourself?"

"About ... myself? Well...."

That lad is going to be a whale of a doctor.

The human essence is delicate, precious, to be nurtured tenderly and with love. Does not healing the spirit fall within a physician's purview?

To Hear or Not to Hear

For ten years I worked with third-year medical students, mostly focusing on interviewing skills. Over and over I observed people talking *at* each other: doctor at bewildered patient, mother at sullen daughter. Communicating with another person means listening with attention and respect. This skill turns out to be remarkably difficult to teach.

Have you ever known a married couple who, when with other people, never hear each other? One roars off in a dozen directions unrelated to what his or her spouse might be saying? She tramps all over the punch line to his joke; he plows a furrow smack through her account of a tender moment. I've known people who have been married for years and operate like that, yet neither takes obvious offense. I prefer not to imagine what Barbara would have said if I had followed even one of their examples. Then add another layer: deafness.

Ada and Nils always came to see me together. After fifty-three years of marriage, they indeed had come to look like each other. Or, wait, is it pets who come to resemble masters? Anyway. Nils was a lively seventy-nine; Ada a year younger. I remember one consultation:

I brought my chair to face them. "So, what brings the Bensons to the office today?" I chirped.

"Nice place you got here, Doc," Nils said.

"Thank you, we've just repainted. What—"

"Doc, don't see no way we could be related."

Ada roared, "Speak up, Nils. Doc can't make sense of you when you mutter like that."

Nils said, "Not even on my mother's side. She was a Johnson, ya know."

I said, "I just need to know who the patient is today."

"As far's I know, Doc, the patent's still good. Them Johnsons the best outboard motors ever invented."

"No, no, Nils, I need to know who's sick today."

"Gosh, Doc, I don't never wear nothin' made out of silk. 'Tain't practical up here where it gets so dang cold."

Ada said, "You gotta speak up, Doc. Cain't hear what you're sayin'. Too soft a voice."

I raised my output by thirty decibels. "I assume one of you has a medical problem."

"Nothin' wrong with my ass, Doc," Nils informed me, God, and half the people in the waiting room. "My bowels work better'n the dang alarm clock."

Ada bellowed, "Why you interested our cows, Doc? Thought you was strict-like a people doc!"

Nils shouted, "Nothing wrong my peeing, either. Once I get 'er goin', comes good as a hose."

I hollered, "I have an idea. Let's conduct this interview by exchanging written notes, since it's so hard for you to hear me."

"Hell, Doc, I ain't afeared of you."

Ada said, "Nils, you never told me you got bit. Where?"

Huh?

I scribbled frantically and then passed over a sheet of paper. It read, "Who is sick, and how?"

Nils roared, "Doc, can you write that in Norwegian?"

Ada screamed, "Nils, how come you want Doc to bite you? Don't sound sanitary."

I shouted, "Ada, no one is planning to bite anyone. I just need to know—"

Nils piped up, "All you gotta do is ask, Doc."

I snatched back the paper to add, "Don't you two think it would be a good idea to get hearing aids?"

Ada dug reading glasses from her purse and peered over them at my hen scratchings. She grinned coyly. Yes, dang it, *coyly*.

"You should learn how to write so's a body could tell what you're sayin', Doc. And those hearing gadgets? If Nils and I could hear each other, our lives wouldn't be near as interestin'."

The Boman Incident

MINNESOTA'S LAST FRONTIER was Koochiching County, across Rainy River from Canada. Pioneers lived by different standards than we do today; toughness earned more respect than did fine manners. Legendary Old Doc Rowland, with his bear-like behavior, belonged to that era.

His house had become a hospital the way dust collects on a windowsill: gradually, without anyone intending it or even realizing it was happening. An overnight patient here, a woman in labor there. Doc lived and practiced in Kenmore, a small town sixty miles from Northpine. I knew of him, for tales of his exploits wafted about the countryside like ghosts out of some Irish fantasy. Despite how often our spoors crossed, I never actually met him. Odd, given how entwined our careers became for a while.

Periodically, demon rum seduced Old Doc.

Nurse Sarah had worked for him for thirty years. Knowing his moods, she steered him to his disheveled basement apartment when he was no longer functioning, then called me.

"Doc's indisposed right now, Dr. Mac, and uh—"

"The brandy flu?"

"Well. . . ."

"What do you need?"

She'd say, "Mrs. Jones is in the hospital with pneumonia," or

"Joe Johnson bust his leg," or ... you get the idea. I'd sigh, she'd chuckle, I'd ask when.

One evening at about eight o'clock Sarah called. "A woman in labor and Doc's—you know. Could you? Would you?"

In 1949, I had not grasped the majesty of the word "No."

Obstetrics is the most unpredictable part of medicine. Run and wait. I arrived at Doc's "hospital" and examined the patient. She was undeniably in labor, had had six babies already, was dilated halfway. Dang. A wild trip back to Northpine would probably result in a backseat delivery. Nurse Sarah and I settled down to wait. Sight of us relaxing in the corner seemed to influence the mother-to-be: she went to sleep.

Sarah apologized. Again. My streak of Irish volatility bowed to my Scottish stoicism, and I sighed. Sarah started talking about Doc and his ways.

"He isn't always drunk, Dr. Mac."

"Just at inconvenient—Sure."

"I din't never meet anyone set out to get hooked on the sauce."

"Yeah, me either."

"A lotta people think Doc's kind of a hopeless old fart."

I was to disagree?

"They talk about yankin' his license," Sarah said, "stuff like that. Thing is, most of the time he really tries. Who else would take care of our people around here? He's been alone for forty-five years. No other doctor to talk to, help out. He's saved a ton a lives by bein' here, and when there was no chance, he'd sit by a bedside more nights'n you can count, holdin' a hand, soothin' someone scared of dying."

I was tempted to launch into a self-righteous declamation,

but I made the mistake of looking earnest, gray-haired Sarah straight in the eye. She read me, and I zipped up.

"He's a *person*, Dr. Mac, same as you and me, and even though he ain't perfect, well, he's stayed on here all these years. More'n anyone else, *I* know how much he cares and how hard he tries when he ain't—when he doesn't let—"

I patted Sarah's hand. "I hear you."

She blew her nose with a honk to shame a lumberjack. "Think Doc don't have feelin's? I want to tell you something 'bout him. I'm the only one knows the whole story, 'cause I was there. See...."

"The whole town buzzed over the Boman thing," Sarah explained. "Oh, I doubt that anyone saw things different. Doc's friends said 'So what?' and everyone else just shook their heads and said 'What next?' Ain't that the way life is?

"Doc received a letter on November the second, 1929," nurse Sarah continued. "Ain't a date I'm likely to forget. See, Doc never sent out bills, and he received most payments cash in hand. The amount a mail he got in a year was a light load.

Doc's letter came from Detroit. "Hardly the kind of place where a body would know anyone," said Sarah. "The address on the front was wrote in beautiful rounded letters out of some penmanship class: Dr. Theodore Rowland, M D, Kenmore, Minnesota. Down in the left lower corner it read, Please Forward If Necessary. On the back was a return address: T. Geddes, some street in Detroit, Michigan.

"I was changin' linen of Old Man Styles's bed. You can see through the doorway to Doc's little office from there. He was sorta pushin' that letter around on his desk, like it had spooked him someway. He wiped his hands on his pants, picked up the envelope, cut the flap with his pen knife, and read the letter.

"After a minute, he shoved it aside. He reached for the brandy bottle he kept in a cubbyhole of his desk and drank it straight down."

The expectant mother stirred and licked her lips. Nurse Sarah bobbed up and moistened them with a damp cloth. "Better wait for a drink of water," she said, her voice soothing as a honey cordial. She patted the woman's shoulder, then returned to sit beside me.

"Clara Boman was an old hand at this birthing business," Sarah explained, "what with eight kids already packed into that dinky Boman shack. Clara began to labor early on November third, and she showed up here about 5:00 AM. Minnie was the nurse working that night. She allowed to Clara as how Doc was on the premises all right, though a mite indisposed with the flu.

"'I'll fetch him; give me time, Clara,' Minnie hollered.

"'Won't be long!' Clara yelled back.

"Minnie was accustomed to Doc's bouts of brandy-flavored flu and was good at fillin' in the gaps. Still, doctorin' *is* best done by doctors. She told me she bounced down and up them stairs to his basement apartment three, four times during the next ten minutes, trying to fetch Doc, until she was as out of breath as Clara, her tryin' so hard to hold back." Sarah grinned at me suddenly. "Be good iffen you docs had some experience at what *that's* like," she said. I wrinkled my nose and returned her smile.

"Finally Clara hollered to Minnie, 'It's a comin'!'—and there it was. A boy, squawking at the top of his lungs. Everything went fine, of course, just the way God intended.

"'Bout then, Doc recovered from his 'flu' to some extent, and he shuffled on the scene just as Minnie was deliverin' the afterbirth.

"He poked at Boy Boman. 'Kid.'

"'Hi, Doc,' Clara Boman said. 'Thank God you was here. We got such faith in you we wouldn't want no one else.'

"Minnie rolled up her eyes, but not where Doc could see her.

"'Kid,' Doc repeated. He poked again, and Boy Boman screwed up to cry.

"'Maybe you could sign the birth certificate, Doc,' Minnie said, busy with those things that have to be done after a woman makes a mess all over from havin' a baby.

"Right about here is where things took a turn off track. Doc wrapped the baby in a receiving blanket, tucked him under one arm like a loaf of French bread, and headed back down to his quarters. Minnie was so startled she just stared after the spot where he disappeared. She ran to the head of the stairs in time to hear him set the lock of the door to his rooms.

"Dr. Mac, you gotta understand how things were back then. There weren't any trained nurses for a hundred miles. Minnie was a nurse because Doc *said* she was. Having six kids of her own, there was no one around better qualified. She had worked for Doc for ten years and was used to certain hospital routines. This for damn sure was not one of them. She stayed his senior employee 'counta she never talked back or questioned orders, for Doc could explode faster than anyone you'd want to meet.

"Clara Boman remained unawares, looking forward to her day of rest before heading home to the chaos of her lively family. Minnie put her to bed, then tiptoed downstairs to listen at the apartment door. Boy Boman's baby talk seemed usual. Of Doc there was no sound.

"Anxious and puzzled, she crept back upstairs to deal with Old Man Styles, Clara, and the others. About that time, Woody arrived from his café, bringin' breakfasts for the patients.

"Minnie peered into the Campbell's Soup carton he plunked on her desk.

"'Bacon and eggs *again*. Can't you try something else occasionally?'

"'It's easy and *your* customers ain't regulars, 'cepting Old Man Styles.'

"'Well, everything curdles into grease in a hurry.'

"'Then quit your bellyaching and get to passing it around.'

"Minnie picked up two chipped porcelain plates and headed for the front room. Between stokin' the three wood stoves that heated the place, collectin' lardy dishes, and reportin' to me, her daytime replacement, she kinda forgot her concern.

"Me, I was new at bein' a designated nurse, didn't know all Doc's routines. Still, bein' young and full a ginger, I decided to fret, thinking 'Someone really should do something' and 'What will the mother think?'

"When Clara Boman asked me about her new son, I said 'He's fine. He's—fine.'

"'When can I see him? My milk's startin' to come in.'

"'Well, look, you'll have him for the next eighteen years. Uh—The latest theory—Pretend you're chargin' up your batteries, sort of. Yeah, that's it.'

"'Never thought of it that way. A grand idea.'

"The day wore on. When I rapped at Doc's door, he'd growl, 'Go away.' About three thirty in the afternoon, Edna arrived to begin her tour of duty. I dragged her down them basement steps, and together we banged on Doc's door. The racket woke Boy Boman, and he began to holler. Doc rumbled, 'Tarnation.'

"'Please, sir,' I said, 'we thought maybe we should—The baby hasn't been bathed—He may be hungry.'

"'Tarnation,' Doc said again.

"'Sir, we could take him upstairs. His mother probably would like to see him.'

"'Go away,' Doc growled. 'Wait. Get me a bottle of milk. And diapers.'

"'Sir, why don't you just let us do that for you? It's properly—'

"'No.'

"'—women's work—'

"'Get the bottle!'

"'—and the Lord's plan. Edna, maybe you'd best fetch a bottle and some diapers.'

"Edna, being youthful and having no kids at all, bounded up them stairs two at a time.

"When Doc opened the door a crack and grabbed the supplies, I peeked as far as I could, regular periscope eyes, but all I saw was the customary litter of his room. Boy Boman made suckling noises and snorts of gratitude when he stopped drinkin' long enough to breathe.

"The door had been firmly locked again; I tried it ever so carefully.

"Things came to a head the next morning. Minnie, Edna, Tillie, and I were Rowland Hospital's staff. Minnie stayed on after her night shift, and we met as a group about 9:00 AM.

"I started. 'I say it's time we have to do something. I say call in the law.'

"'Constable Todd Windner?' said Minnie.

"'I know, but who else is there?'

"I marched into Doc's office and liked to crank the handle

off the phone. Operator Clarice Odegaard was tart when she answered.

"'Get me Todd Windner. A law matter. Sort of. Maybe.'

"While I waited, my gaze slid across the commotion that was Doc's desk. A letter lay open on it. I read it, couldn't stop once I'd started. When Todd answered, I had a time remembering what I wanted."

"That silly goose, constable Todd Windner, arrived, once he'd run outta made-up excuses not to. He blinked at me like a daytime owl. 'Let's get this straight,' he says. 'You want me to bust in Doc's door, to his own room, in his own hospital, 'cause he's taking care of a baby, by hisself?'

"'Well, yes.'

"'I ain't sure that's legal. God Almighty, what if a constable busts the law?'

"I shook my head, stubborn-like. 'There's a baby in there and we should find out—shouldn't we?'

"Todd's lip trembled, and he touched the badge clipped to his jacket. When he walked down the stairs to Doc's basement room, he held firmly to the handrails. He wiped his palms on his uniform pants and stared at the door as though the devil hisself would leap out if he opened it. He made a knocker of his finger and tapped the door's wooden panel. Boy Boman whimpered.

"'Who's there?' Doc growled.

"Todd squeaked like a boy soprano. 'It's the law, Doc. Sir. Todd. Constable Windner.'

"'Tarnation.'

"'Open the door, sir. Please.'

"'Go away.'

"'I can't, sir. I gotta see—You have a baby in there.' There was no response. 'Sir, I'll be forced to break in this-here door. Please open up.' Silence.

"Todd tried the handle. The door was unlocked. He pushed gingerly; it swung wide.

"Doc sat on a wooden rung chair beside his chest of drawers. The second drawer from the bottom had been pulled out to serve as a cradle. He held a bottle delicately in those huge fingers of his while Boy Boman sucked in the natural way of a hungry infant.

"Minnie and I crept into Doc's room to peer over Todd's shoulder. Minnie sidled to the drawer and lifted Boy Boman tenderly. She flushed, glanced at Doc, and said, 'Mrs. Boman wants to go home.' She scurried up the stairs.

"Doc shook the empty bottle and set it carefully on top of the chest. I reached into my pocket and slid out a letter, folded on its creases. I laid it on the table beside Doc's easy chair. I sniffled and for a moment damn near patted Doc on the shoulder. I ducked my head and trotted upstairs.

"That letter? I'll never forget it. It said:

Dear Daddy:

I feel strange writing that, because I don't ever remember saying it. To me you are only an old picture I still have around here. I don't know if you want to know that you are now a grandfather. There, I've told you, and you are. Tyson, he's my husband, had no objection, and for some reason I wanted to name our son Theodore.

I hope this finds you well. And that you don't mind.
Sincerely, your loving daughter,
Thelma

· · ·

Doc and Sarah both died decades ago, yet their story remains among my most poignant memories. Her earnest plea for compassion was an early prod to my own search for wisdom and that grace known as maturity. I was the brash neophyte filled with the latest pronouncements of medical school experts, convinced that I knew "how medicine should be practiced." But certainty when it comes to science must always be tempered, for new discoveries often shoot gaping holes in cherished dogma. For me at that time, such awareness lay years and painful life experiences ahead.

Any physician worth his or her salt has accepted the risk of failure in daring to treat fellow humans. I believe it is a greater sin to do nothing in the name of fearful self-protection than it is to make a mistake. No doctor-patient encounter is exempt from the possibility of error. Such is a healer's responsibility. As Sarah said, "Doc was there and he tried." Far more often than not, he succeeded.

I wonder: who will be *my* judge?

Ardith

ARDITH WAS FORTY-EIGHT that day she sat quietly in my office, her features somber. She was neatly dressed, as usual, and her hair had been done in a functional cut and style, consistent with her role as a nurse. The Ardith I knew from regular contact at the hospital exuded cheer and combined skill with nurturing—vitamins for the souls of bedridden patients. On extended leave from work, she was missed by staff and patient alike.

How long had it been since her husband had died? Four months? So abrupt, dead in bed. At fifty, a man might expect a higher number from inscrutable nature's lottery.

Now Ardith wore the yoke of those "why" questions, of grief in its myriad incarnations.

I leaned forward. "How are you coming?"

Her response was delayed, like a conversation between moon and earth. "Coming?"

"Losing a spouse is considered one of the most traumatic events a person can endure."

"Maybe I have cancer or ... something."

"Not according to all those tests we put you through last month."

"Maybe I'm ... not worth...."

"Ah."

She opened her purse, peered into it, shut it again.

"Would you care to tell me what it has been like these past months?" I asked.

Again the delayed response. "Hell cannot be any worse than ... some things here on earth."

"Tell me."

She looked about vaguely. "Alone. Lethargy, until it comes time to go to bed. Then my heart pounds and I can't catch my breath. I stumble out to a chair in the living room, sit up until dawn."

I chewed the inside of my lip. "Ardith, have you been considering suicide?"

Delay. "If I have?"

"I would feel obligated to send you to a hospital where attendants could make certain that you didn't."

"You think I'm crazy."

"I think you have suffered a great loss. I'm concerned because, frankly, you seem stuck somewhere in the grief process. I see you slipping into depression. I wouldn't have predicted that you were a candidate. Still, grief is a powerful emotion."

"And guilt," she whispered.

"Guilt?"

"I should have just said no."

"I don't understand."

Her sigh stretched the limit of a breath. "He was using those pills you prescribed for his heart, beta-blockers. The thing is...."

She opened her purse again. I handed her a box of tissues.

"He had become impatient with the side effects. You understand."

"Perhaps," I said, "but it's okay to be specific."

She studied a sodden, shredded tissue. "Here I am, a nurse, and you're a doctor, yet I'm having as much trouble explaining as though I were some naïve bride."

I patted her hand. "My Ojibwe friends tell me that, in the old culture, if a person wanted to say something difficult, he or she just puked it out. Saved time."

She reached for the box of tissues again. "It kept him from ... he said he couldn't ... couldn't maintain an erection."

I nodded. "Not uncommon. Some choice." I waited.

"He told me he had quit taking the pills. Then ... that night ... he wanted to make love and ... I should have just said no!"

"Did it happen while you were—"

"Yes! Oh God, RAM, right there in the middle of ... he just collapsed and ... I tried the CPR we practice at the hospital. It didn't work!"

I waited while she cried. Then I said, "Let's look at guilt for a minute. Were you responsible for his stopping the pills?"

"No, I suppose not, but if I had realized ... he could have tapered off. Isn't that what you usually recommend?"

I looked at her.

She sighed again. "That night, when he asked if we could ... you know, I didn't say no, then. . . ." She yanked out another tissue.

I asked, "If you try to be responsible for more than yourself, how does that work?"

She bowed her head; a lock of hair fell across her face.

"What do you think we could do to take this burden off your shoulders?"

She shrugged, hope not even a ghostly glimmer in her eyes. "I had no chance to say good-by. To say how sorry I am."

"Would you like to do that now?"

For an instant the look in her eye branded me a lunatic.

"Let's try," I said. I drew curtains across the windows and turned off the bright medical-office lights. I pulled an empty chair to face her and placed mine beside hers.

"Close your eyes," I suggested.

"What is this?"

"If Joe were sitting on this other chair, and you knew you had half an hour to tell him those things you regret having left unsaid, what would they be?"

"Doctor!"

"Try. And relax, the way you would have spoken to him."

She closed her eyes, but her back was stiff as an ironing board. "This is silly."

"Eyes closed, now. He's on the chair. Waiting...."

"Joe?" She dabbed with Kleenex. "Are you really there? What would I have... maybe I didn't let you know how much... how dear you were. Are. Have always been. Busyness! Job and church and all those volunteer activities. Love changes as years go by, becoming a comfortable mantle, even though a touch of your hand still...."

At last she whispered, "Good-by, Joe. Thanks for... everything."

I waited while final tears dried on her cheeks. She looked up at me, as though surprised to find I was sitting beside her.

"He understood," she said. "He's that way. Now I believe I'll be able to sleep again."

I didn't trust my voice, so I just nodded. We stood. She started for the door, looked over a shoulder, and held out her arms. My back creaked from the intensity of her hug.

Joel Monroe

M ANY HAVE ASKED whether I was ever in physical danger from a delusional patient. Such things happen, although rarely. Two physician acquaintances of mine each had the experience of finding a gun-toting psychotic at the front door. Both prevailed in the situations, and no one was hurt.

A rough calculation convinces me that over the course of my career I had six or seven hundred thousand patient encounters. My word. Out of those, exactly twice was I "threatened" by a psychotic patient.

The first came during a house call. A man was experiencing an acute psychotic break with reality. Upon my arrival, I had given him an injection of a neuroleptic drug, a formula that helps break the bonds of delusion and hallucination. I dragged a chair beside the bed to monitor the effects. Suddenly, he leaped out of bed, knocked me to the floor, sat astride me, and squeezed my throat, rumbling, "The radio told me to kill you." I have never been much of a warrior, but panic is a magnificent energizer. I broke free, ran for help, and with police assistance was able to sedate him more completely. The poor man, a gentle soul when himself, apologized abjectly once he returned from treatment.

A second incident occurred on my own territory.

· · ·

I was at my desk wading through charts when assistant Elaine Andresen knocked at my office door and stepped through the slight opening. "He's here!" she squeaked.

I adopted a visage of patient forbearance, tented fingertips before my face. "*He* is a fairly indeterminate pronoun, although it serves to eliminate slightly more than half the human race."

"That guy!"

I said pompously, "A fact of some definitive value, but *guy* isn't a great deal better."

"The one—St. Louis—last May—psychologist—"

I smiled benignly. "Now we're—"

My blood froze. I had heard the expression; that's exactly how it felt. "He's *here?*"

Elaine was nearly crying. "That's what I'm trying to tell you."

"That *guy?*"

"Joel Monroe."

"My God." I experimented with an array of primitive reflexes: sprinting pulse, harsh breathing, sweaty palms, tremors.

She said, "He's pacing out there in the waiting room, from the green chair to the fish tank, around the—He's all pale and his eyes look funny and he's muttering to himself and—RAM, I'm scared!"

"No need to be, I—hope. How big is he?"

She measured the air before her face, held her hand level with her forehead. "So, maybe...." She moved her hand higher.

"I wish I remembered him."

"Doctor, how could you forget?"

"Not *about* him. I just don't remember what he looks like."

What to do? Without his chart in hand, I could not recall why he had consulted me back in mid-May, at the opening of fishing season. Joel Monroe was a high school psychologist from St. Louis, Missouri. He had sent me the first letter in July, apparently in response to a routine statement of medical charges. It consisted of seventeen pages of handwritten vituperation, incoherent collages of words and phrases, all with the theme that he, Joel Monroe, was "perturbed with one R. A. MacDonald, who classifies himself as a doctor, although the use of MD is itself fraught with question when one is not present to see the bread come out of the oven."

He went on to detail his displeasure that "aforesaid individual who claims to the estate of physician-hood and masquerades as a noble healer would dare to charge him for any care delivered, however recklessly, in May of this very year." The letter ended with the following diatribe: "retribution is more appropriate than recompense, but in the frightful event that payment becomes inevitable, I will forthrightly make restitution, vile and unwise though it be, and if that is insufficient, I will personally see that you receive your dues—ghastly mess!— in hamburgers. That, buddy, is a hell of a lot of hamburgers."

For the past month I had received such epistles at the rate of one or two a week. I had long since reached a diagnosis of paranoid schizophrenia. "Doesn't anyone in St. Louis notice?" I had grumped to Barbara. "Maybe I should call his school."

"It's summer," she reminded me.

"Great. Psychiatric advice from a psychotic psychologist."

"Sooner or later," she had said.

Well, sooner was now. I opened the bottom desk drawer and rummaged through its nearly forgotten odds and ends. Aha, the blackjack. My predecessor had told me I might need it sometime, although I think he had envisioned my using it on a rambunctious lumberjack rather than on a mixed-up psychologist. I held up the leather-covered weapon for Elaine's inspection.

She said, "RAM, whatever do you plan to do?"

I pulled the client chair to the end of my desk and set it facing mine. The sap I placed in the top drawer, open enough that I could lay hand on it directly. I chuckled sardonically. "If that poor joker reaches for a handkerchief or something, *pow!* Goose egg. Show him in. And Elaine, if you hear any commotion in here at all, call Louie from the village police department."

Elaine's round-eyed agitation left no doubt that she considered me to be as certifiable as my patient.

Joel Monroe crept into the office. He turned out to be a plump, balding, nondescript little man whose appearance triggered no memory. Sweat speckled his skin; limp hair straggled across his pate, disturbed by the vague explorations of his restless hands. His head jerked from side to side, and his gaze darted up, down, from me back to the door, just closing on Elaine's terrified face. He took a tentative step and repeated his lightning inspection of me and my surroundings.

I extended a hand cautiously. What was protocol for greeting a psychotic who had invested so much energy into personal threats? The man ignored my gesture and instead slunk to the chair I had arranged so carefully. What did they say in shoot-'em-up shows? Watch his hands.

"What—" I brought my voice to a lower register. "What can I do for you, sir?"

The man gaped at me and his lip trembled. He said, "I—I—don't know." More sweat appeared on his skin, like dew on a cool morning. His tongue darted along his lips. "I was here—" He jerked his head to look over a shoulder. "I should—Now, you're Doctor—"

Joel Monroe leaped from his chair and vanished into the hallway like a sprinter out of the blocks. I bolted to the waiting room, that stupid blackjack, seized in the convulsion of the man's departure, dangling from my fingers, in time to see him streak across the lawn to a car at the curb. He left as though the custodians of hell were on his heels. Who can say that they weren't?

"Elaine," I called, "ring the highway patrol while I reach the county welfare office."

I plowed through the bureaucracy of the welfare department. Speaker number three proved to be executive director Thaddeus Bumfry.

"The man is sick," I explained.

"Did he attack you?" asked Director Bumfry.

"No, but all those letters, his appearance—"

"What psychological tests have you performed?"

"Tests! Good Lord."

"No MMPI, no Rorschach, nothing objective?"

"Mr. Bumfry, we were never on that level of communication."

"You say he's from St. Louis. Missouri? Not the county?"

"Correct."

"Then clearly he is not our problem."

"But—"

"If we commit him here in Minnesota, assuming that your speculations are correct, look at what it would cost us. Once we start something like that, no matter where he's from, we're stuck."

"The man's sick."

"We can all hope that Mr. Monroe won't stop until he passes the Iowa border."

"I don't believe this."

"I'd advise cancellation of your pick-up request to the state patrol. The problem of a charge, you see."

"But—"

"It's been good to talk to you, Dr. MacDonald. We were discussing at the county commissioners' meeting just the other day what a good job you're doing for our clients in your area."

"Holy buckets."

"Feel free to call anytime. That's what we're here for."

"Doesn't anyone care?"

The phone hummed at me in the key of C major.

The letters ceased. Maybe someone finally noticed. In his case, as in so many others for a physician with a large contingent of tourists-patients, that final chapter is missing. A mystery.

Harvey and Frances

W E WHO SURVIVE to the Octobers of life are made of special sinews and bone. Though skin that once fit snugly
may lie in wrinkles, the person it encloses feels essentially the
same as he or she did during vibrant youth. So, what is aging?
Not necessarily physical deterioration: Dr. Hawking, the remarkable cosmologist trapped in a body ravaged by ALS—Lou
Gehrig's Disease—remains the same source of insights into our
universe that he was when he could still form words with his
lips and larynx. Erosion of the brain, perhaps? When the brain
goes, so leaks away personality, companion, lover, expert in the
life it once controlled. To anticipate this theft of personhood, to
be aware of its happening, is as terrifying as being a passenger
strapped in an airplane hurtling toward earth, knowing but
helpless.

Harvey and Frances were patients, and friends.

Harvey had been an executive, important to his company.
He chose to retire at age sixty-two and moved to Northpine so
that he could enjoy in health the area he regarded as heaven on
earth. His gnarled Viking features were made handsome by dint
of the zest he held for life. And his wife, Frances: she was a vibrant, bubbly, slender creature who could have leaped out of
some Disney fantasy. She exuded cheer and love: person-to-
person love that was never flirtatious. She gardened, she sang

in the Church of Christ choir, she ran—and not with that grim, sour determination I see on the faces of most who dash past as I stroll through life, but with abandon, like a colt delighting in the fact that it can.

Both of them enriched our community with their intellects and their involvement in the town's affairs. They were a couple blessed—and generous with their blessings.

All the while, Alzheimer's Disease gnawed away the treasures of Harvey's mind.

As terrifying as looming dementia is to a victim aware of its coming, the spouse of such a patient shoulders burdens unimaginable during the partnership years of a marriage. When I look into the eyes of an Alzheimer patient, I see confusion, wistful pleading, anxiety, and the restlessness of one who senses self-determination leaching away. When I look deep into the eyes of a loving caregiver, I see despair, guilt over anger impossible to deny, and fatigue from endless night vigils as the demented spouse wanders deeper into chaos. I never decided which fate seemed the worse.

Frances came to see me one dark day, exhausted, her brightness dimmed. She could no longer care for Harvey, feared that he would fall, or escape during his delirious nightly wanderings, or set their home on fire. They moved into a place that offered assisted living.

I had not seen Harvey or Frances for a while. When life plows a straight furrow, we so often follow where it leads without stepping aside. Then, the activity director of the housing complex where Harvey and Frances lived called to see if the small jazz group with which I sometimes played would provide music at a dance for the residents. Frustrated musicians, especially jazz aficionados, never turn down a gig, so we in the band agreed.

Harvey and Frances arrived at the activity lounge where the dance would be held. Harvey wore his tuxedo proudly, and Frances's long, dark dress sleekly highlighted her form, which evoked the muscled power of a lean panther. Harvey offered her his arm and for a precious while it was not obvious that she was his lifeline. I stepped away from the band to greet them and help them find seats where they could watch those capable of dancing.

The music picked me up on soaring pinions, and I became only dimly aware of anything beyond the scroll of my fiddle. Then I looked up.

In the center of the small dance area, surrounded by admiring couples in moth-balled finery, Harvey stood like a proud Maypole. Frances spun around him, feet twinkling, skirt swirling, exuding grace and merriment and delight and even, yes, joy! Harvey set aside the vacuous mask his face had become to beam and glide about on sure feet, his gaze never leaving hers. We in the band serenaded Harvey and his bride of forty-five years. Frances threw back her head and her laughter ignited a fire storm of exuberance among the rest of us, we who were ensnared by cold reason and its constraints.

Music has some special resonance for the demented. My wife Jackie and I see evidence of this when we play a few songs in a local nursing home—popular tunes from the twenties and thirties, a jig or a reel. As we play, I see heads that had been drooping listlessly straighten erect and vacant eyes light up. A palsied foot taps the footrest of a wheelchair, and scratchy voices join the melodies floating about the dayroom. It is as though a long-muted inner ear awakens to a familiar tune.

I understood that one day I would minister to Harvey, to the bedridden husk he would become, but I shall always see him as he was that night, leaping free from torment's bonds, if only for a moment, under the enchantment of music.

Oh, Those Office Calls!

A PRIMARY-CARE PHYSICIAN spends more than 80 percent of his working time in the office. In truth, it becomes his second home. Cases included in a generalist's practice are like the quilt I won at a raffle one year: variety in myriad colors and shapes.

.   .   .

Photographer Casey Flanagan was on an assignment for *National Geographic*. A group of latter-day voyageurs was retracing the canoe route of the hardy men who had transported furs from Canada's Northwest Territories to Grand Portage on the shore of Lake Superior some two hundred years before. At times Flanagan and his comrades waded through water too shallow to float a fully loaded canoe. They coped with a rapid flow and rocks slippery as greased bowling balls. He fell and broke a wrist.

His arm showed the typical deformity of what doctors term a "Colle's wrist fracture." Treatment includes restoration of bony anatomy, capturing a suitable position in a plaster cast—and six week's worth of rest.

Flanagan and I discuss options in the refined fashion employed by a pair of Celts resolving any difference of opinion. (Censors will have deleted details: suffice to say, I am losing the negotiation.)

"No more *paddling*," I say for the seventeenth time.

Flanagan explains the historical imperatives driving their mission, well punctuated with finger language.

"I weep in compassion," I scream. Well, declare firmly.

"I'm going anyway!"

"You blockheaded Irish—" There is more, of course, but I draw the curtain of refinement.

What can I do?

It happens that the man in charge of hospital maintenance is a resourceful fellow named Clarence. (No institution can function without someone like him: unflappable, fixes anything.) We consult.

He helps me apply the cast to Flanagan's broken wrist, and I incorporate a concoction of Clarence's into the cast's palmar surface. The idea is that our intrepid Irishman can finish his canoe trip by snuggling the end of the paddle into Clarence's heavy-gauge sheet metal invention. It occurs to me that this device might be considered an anachronism, bringing into question the authenticity of the trek. Would a real voyageur have found a Clarence along the way?

I've wondered how the son-of-a-gun's wrist turned out. The doctor part of me hopes it wasn't crooked after it healed, but that Celtic fire buried deep in me genes can't escape a wee spot o' relish at the thought that Flanagan's middle finger may point a bit to port these days.

. . .

Northpine enjoyed the mystique of not a single town drunk but an entire club of them. Ferdie was a charter member. Village cop Louie Wagenknect brought him to see me one day; the man would never have thought to seek medical care on his own.

"Found him stretched out flat on his belly in the park," Louie said. "On the grass beside the picnic tables. When I got him onto his feet, he kept shaking his head every few seconds—There, like that."

Ferdie demonstrated again. A vigorous twitch, resembling the way my spaniel used to clear himself of water.

"What's happening, Ferdie?" I asked.

"Won't quit," he muttered. Another shake.

"What won't—"

"My ear!"

Ah.

I peeked into Ferdie's right ear canal with my trusty otoscope—and dang near dropped it! Enlarged to "in-your-face" size by the instrument's lens, half a dozen leechlike critters humped busily across Ferdie's eardrum. Freeloaders picked up during his sojourn on Northpine's green sward. I syringed out the blighters—possibly a species of nematodes, according to our entomologist daughter—and made a silent vow to wear combat boots the next time I visited the village recreation area.

It is a secret ambition of doctor-types to have a disease named after them. Since most ailments have already been claimed, there is little wiggle room for us latecomers. Ferdie's situation seems rife with possibilities: Oto-tympanic leechitis (or, maybe, nematoditis) dextro-auriculus MacDonaldi. I can see it now: my own chapter in *Harrison's Principles of Internal Medicine*. Let me know what you think.

· · ·

Angelina arrived at my office bearing signs and symptoms of a cold. I examined her and found no secondary infection.

"I want a shot of penicillin," she mumbled around a wad of Kleenex.

"Antibiotics don't help a cold," I explained.

"Everyone says they do. Give me a shot."

"No, no, you don't understand. Antibiotics kill certain *bacteria* that cause *some* infections but—"

"Are you going to give me a shot?"

"—but they have no effect—"

"I'm in a hurry."

"—on a virus. Therefore—"

"No shot?"

"Uh, no shot."

"Well!"

Angelina departed at a brisk trot. She slammed the front door of my office with such vigor that its glass pane shattered, the shards flying clear back to Margaret's reception desk.

A doctor does have a duty to educate people about medical— Oh, never mind.

. . .

Cerumen, earwax, is a natural secretion that in some individuals collects abundantly and can harden to the consistency of a crayon. It can usually be syringed free using warm water. Not my favorite office event, but a common one. In fact, my very first patient in Northpine was a fellow who came to have his ears cleaned out.

Curriculum around a university medical school appropriately tends to emphasize the kinds of cases that fill an ivory-tower hospital. As a consequence, though, the details of ordinary problems—chicken pox, plantar warts, sore throats, earwax—are ignored.

Dear friend, nurse Leola, handed me an ear syringe that first morning. I had never seen one before and was as uneasy at its size as was the patient. I could have been persuaded that it was meant to inject a horse. I didn't have a clue how to use it. Leola did the job, earning me my first two-dollar fee.

She let me watch, though.

. . .

Joe Sattersmoen arrived at my office complaining of hearing loss in his right ear, a stuffy feeling, even a touch of vertigo. Earwax, case number seven hundred, I grumped silently. I took up my otoscope, but... earwax *never* sports wings. I syringed a full-grown, inch-long moth from his ear canal. Some people must sleep more soundly than I.

. . .

Five-year-old Bridgit McTaggert was one of those sprites who could convince a man that Ireland lies just beyond the nearest grove of pines. I think it's the eyes—a shade of green, a sparkle denied most of us. Her mother, Colleen, had brought her to the office for a minor childhood affliction, something that did not shatter the precarious empathy a doctor tries to maintain with those citizens who are less than three feet tall.

Colleen was a deputy sheriff, as cheerful an officer as I've known. At the end of the visit, she grinned, gathered up jackets, and took her daughter's hand. "Thanks, Doc. Well, back to work. I've got a handful of subpoenas to serve."

I followed them to the waiting room doorway and heard the lass burble to those assembled, "Guess what? My mom—she— Mom has to go and serve penises."

. . .

Mrs. Jameson was seven months pregnant. In 1952, ultrasound as a tool for following a pregnancy was still on a far distant horizon. Gender and most other features of an unborn child were as easy to surmise as they would be by feeling a newborn through a thick, soft pillow, in the dark.

"I'd like an x-ray of the baby," Mrs. Jameson said.

I said, "We have no indication of need for a film. Your baby is the right size and in a normal position, verified by palpation through your abdominal wall. We don't want to expose you or baby to unnecessary radiation. Why do you ask?"

"I wanted to see what color its hair is."

.   .   .

The trouble with making an appointment is that a person, not unreasonably, expects it to mean something. But when it's summertime busy, when more than half of a day's patients are tourists who have run afoul of some law of nature or physics, who stagger in at any old time, well, you can imagine what happens to the appointment book.

Ms. X. was one of the latter. Nurse Verna Empey had ushered her past stony-eyed appointees, and with good cause. The patient had been bleeding heavily from the vagina and complained of pain in her lower abdomen. Mr. Y., her escort, looked as worried as she.

I did a cautious pelvic exam and found what appeared to be a considerable tear in her vaginal vault next to the uterine cervix, sealed from bleeding for the moment by a large liver-like clot. I could not predict the extent of the damage. I went to the head of the exam table and studied the pair. "I need to know what happened," I said.

They looked at me like the prisoner does the judge and sighed in unison.

"Okay," Mr. Y. said. "Thing is—God. See, Doctor, we're not

married. We—our spouses were away for the weekend and—well, X and I went camping out in the Boundary Waters Canoe Area Wilderness and when we made love, it hurt her."

I said, "She has torn, how badly, how *deeply*, I can't tell. I must refer her to Duluth, to a specialist capable of coping with a gynecologic emergency."

Ms. X. left by ambulance while Mr. Y. faced a solitary trip back home in his car. I've wondered: how many miles did it take to fashion an explanation certain to hold water?

．　．　．

In 1952, an isolated general practitioner was expected to cover all bases. Radiologists were comfortably ensconced in hospitals one to two hundred miles from Northpine. To obtain a fluoroscopic barium-contrast study of the intestinal tract, in search of ulcers or tumors, meant the patient had to cart his body to a facility on the Iron Range or in Duluth. As Gust Jankowski put it, "Hell no, Doc, I ain't goin' down there. *You* do it."

You do it. The Northpine Hospital had the equipment, my predecessor had performed his own fluoroscopies, I had peered over his shoulder those zillion times—and Gust sat there, giving me the old fish-eyed stare. I sighed, agreeing once more to make a first-time "solo flight."

"Come back tomorrow. Here's what you have to do as preparation for your stomach x-ray."

The following morning, I eased Gust behind the fluoroscopy screen, turned out the overhead light, handed him his barium cocktail, and told him to start drinking. I watched the opaque material slide down his esophagus and plop into a liquid pool in his stomach.

Liquid pool?

"Gust," I squawked, "I told you not to eat breakfast this morning."

"Hell, Doc, I skipped it, just like you said."

"Then—what's in there?"

"Nothin' but a couple little old doughnuts and coffee. Doc, you can't expect a man to starve."

. . .

Little Petey Tannenbaum stuck an M&M candy (a green one) up his nostril (right side). Cissy Tannenbaum was one of those mothers eternally trying to do the right thing yet regularly coming up a second short, as in M&Ms up a three-year-old's nose.

I had devised a gadget for coping with this common class of afflictions. I took apart an old Allis forceps, equipped with paired shallow cups instead of teeth, and used a separated half to ease past the M&M (crayon, pea, bean, Monopoly game token, peanut butter) and gently scoop it free. Worked marvelously, did not traumatize delicate nasal tissues, scared the kid into a frenzy—

There was that.

The challenge of convincing a two- or three-year-old that a doctor has benign intentions was complicated by my unique foreign-body remover, so nearly resembling one of those probes dentists favor. It was hold-the-kid-down-and-get-the-job-done time.

Whew. Cissy Tannenbaum picked up the retrieved M&M.

"I'm going to show this to his *father*. Maybe now Big Pete will understand what a mother has to put up with." More of that sort of thing.

I waved the Tannenbaums toward the waiting room and stepped to Room Two, commiserated with Mrs. Anderson about her arthritis, returned to the hallway, and reached for the chart beside Room Three.

Petey Tannenbaum?

Cissy was apoplectic, arms waving, Jerry Colona eyes glaring. "I get to the waiting room, Josie Smith wants to know what all the fuss is about, I show her the piece of candy, Petey grabs it and shoves it back up his nose! Doctor, make him don't do that!"

Hannah Munson

HANNAH was a daughter of original settler Hiram "Swamp Cougar" Munson. Those pioneers who first came to the Northpine area had arrived on foot, after a hike of one hundred miles through bogs and forests so dense they blocked out the sun. Tough as were the likes of old Hiram, the women they persuaded to come with them, to leave the rough comfort of an 1890s Mesabi Iron Range town, matched them step for sodden step. Hannah's mother, Olga, had been of that stripe. Hiram and Olga felled trees and scraped a living from peat-sour land that had been at the bottom of a vast glacial lake not so many thousands of years before.

In those days, babies pretty much delivered themselves, unless old Mary Bineshi, the Indian midwife from over at Chippewa Lake, happened to be available. Thing was, by the time a runner reached Mary, and by the time they had slogged through all that wilderness to wherever the baby was expected, most likely it was already at its mother's breast.

Hannah was fifty-nine the day she first came to my office. Lines earned from squinting at the sun crisscrossed her face, and winter's harshness had thickened patches of skin. A Ma Kettle with dignity, she wore a dress that extended from a plain collar to an unobtrusive hem at mid-calf. Hannah was of the generation that considered store-bought clothing an extravagant affectation; she sewed her own. I cannot believe that she ever used make-up in her life. The image I drew of her feminine strength could have placed her on the seat of a Conestoga wagon headed west.

She sat beside the desk in my office, her gaze unblinking. She had come alone. In the ethos of her family—old Hiram and her laconic, weather-gnarled husband, Jake—"doctorin'" was women's business, not an affair men involved themselves in except under the direst of circumstances.

She told her story in clipped, blunt terms: weight loss, vague tiredness, an appetite "gone south." Pain? A bit, down in the left flank, "nothin' a body can't stand, Doc." And yes, some constipation, "a little blood on the ass wipe."

I palpated a hard mass in the left side of her abdomen, in the region of the descending colon. Blood tests confirmed the anemia her pallor promised. A barium contrast x-ray study of her large bowel showed the monster that had claimed it: a tumor the size of a grapefruit. I referred Hannah to Duluth, to the care of a surgeon trained in treating cancer.

We doctors are sometimes accused, rightly, of offering more hope than we'd admit to in the privacy of our own thoughts. I'm not sure what the surgeon told Hannah about her prognosis, but I personally had no illusions. When she returned for a follow-up visit at my office a month later, I kept pessimism to myself.

Hannah elected not to return again for about six months. I needed only glance at her to know what I would find from tests I ordered to make it "official." "Come back in a week," I said, "for results of our findings."

Freshly returned from consultations in Duluth, Hannah sank tiredly onto the client chair in my office. On her face I saw the lines chronic pain etches. She braced herself while I inspected the sheaf of medical reports spread before me, checking one more time, inventing delays, wishing, wishing . . . wishing I could at least pass the job to someone else. There was no doubt: Hannah's cancer had spread throughout her body.

I sighed and looked her in the eye.

"I already figured, Doc," she said quietly. "You couldn't keep it from me if you tried. Thank you for what you've done, and those docs in Duluth, too. We-uns 'preciate it, Jake and me."

I gripped her hand, and for the briefest moment she clung.

"Well." She stood and stared out the window of my consultation room, her rugged visage as sturdy as any to grace the prow of a Viking longboat. "There's folks out there," she said, "maybe some a them'll be gone before me. Only difference, they don't know it yet."

Hannah attended the funerals of a neighbor (Stanford, heart attack) and a member of her church (Helen, auto accident) before she was brought to her own memorial. Fate decreed that I should say good-by to this modern-day Valkyrie scant hours before she died. Her head was unbowed.

Marijoan and Foghorn

Both gurneys in our hospital emergency room were occupied. I twitched an eyebrow at nurse Millie.

"Johannsens," she said. "Auto accident. Marijoan's banged up, face and arms, says her shoulder hurts. As for Foghorn, well...."

Oye. "Foghorn" and "emergency room" in the same sentence meant another DWI.

"Are the police here yet?" I asked.

"The sheriff's department is on it. Happened out on County 59, quarter-mile from where they live. Deputy Les Perkins said he'd have to wait until Foghorn sobers up enough to question him, and Marijoan ... well, she's not saying much of anything."

Uh-oh. Head injury? Shock?

I peeked into Foghorn's slot—old beer, and snores to challenge Hedstrom's sawmill—then sidled along the gurney holding Marijoan. She lay quietly on her side. Freckled Norwegian; eyes closed; lips down-turned, tightening at times in gentle moues; graying red hair in haystack disarray. When I touched her shoulder, her lids popped open and she yipped softly.

"Doctor Mac here," I said. "Where do you hurt?"

She studied me, a wild-eyed stare, then subsided. She held out her hands and arms. "Got scratched up, Doc, and I slammed against the door with my shoulder." She raised it gingerly. "Figure those cuts need stitches?"

I peered at an assortment of half- to one-inch incisions. "I'll clean those and close them with a few sutures."

I did my doctor thing: made sure minor wounds weren't distracting attention from more serious injuries. No sign of head, neck, chest, or abdominal damage. A floorboard whack had resulted in a sprained ankle, not uncommon when a car stops abruptly.

Nurse Millie set up a suture tray of sterile supplies and equipment. I dragged a chair next to Marijoan's cot and said, "Fill me in on what happened."

She closed her eyes. I saw that they were scrunching tighter by the moment, and a tear leaked out. She shook her head on its pillow, slowly, a metronome set to some inner torment.

I sighed. "I guess I can connect the dots. Didn't I hear that Foghorn—uh, pardon, Andy—had lost his driver's license?" She chewed her lip hard enough that I began to worry she might bite through it. I said, "Deputy Les Perkins will almost certainly want a blood alcohol, and I'm obligated to draw it for him."

Finally she muttered, "Just sew up my cuts so we can get out of here."

I pulled on rubber gloves and drew lidocaine into a syringe. "I had in mind to keep you the rest of the night. That old 'observation' chestnut, but justified, Marijoan. Anyway, how would we get you both home?"

"I don't want to stay," she whispered.

I readied the anesthetic needle next to one of her cuts and prepared to wield my version of a sewing needle. "I can't tie you in bed, but why not accept a few hours of rest before having to cope with Foghorn's latest...."

I took lack of further objection for acquiescence. After

I finished my tailoring job, Millie trundled her off to bed in Room Three. I sighed and turned my attention to Andrew (Foghorn) Johannsen. All I could detect was profound inebriation.

Later I caught up with Sheriff Perkins. His interview with Foghorn had been of the sputtering variety: "Whad'di do?" "Wha' driver's license?" "I hav'n been drunkin' driv." "Screw you, Dep'y."

Les said, "Odd how things go. Foghorn made it all the way from town, up slippery Basin Crick Road, along County 59 with its coat of compacted snow, 'til he got to the only bare patch on that whole trip, then dang if he didn't go almost straight down into the ditch. Smashed the whole front end of their new car. Go figure." He glanced at a clock. "Doc, let's you and me sign a pact, no more calls 'til morning."

I gave my old comrade a thumb and finger okay, sighed, and returned to the nurses' desk to document what I had just accomplished.

Foghorn was a prototypal Viking: scraggly hair that shade red assumes when passing winters nudge it toward white, a flowing mustache stretched wide above a beard that seemed always four or five days past contact with a razor, a darker auburn than his head hair. His shoulders were like those of a bull moose, arms bigger than my thighs. A brute, some stranger might conclude. The man was as ferocious as a week-old kitten, when sober. His voice was a basso rumble that had earned him his nickname. He was not without a certain charm, if he and beer had been separated long enough. Over the years, I had spent days—well, at least a peck of cumulative hours—trying to convince Foghorn and Marijoan that AA, Al-Anon, and CD treatment were worthwhile. Ever the experienced con man, Foghorn agreed heartily with my suggestions, and that champion of enablers, Marijoan, sat passively through my efforts at persuasion. Any resolve she had built up to help guide him into therapy melted like lard on a hot griddle the moment they got home. Nothing had ever come of my missionary exhortations.

So be it.

I went to see Marijoan on hospital rounds in the morning. She sat propped up in bed, brushing listlessly at a mop of hair damp from the shower. I checked her over and found nothing beyond a burgeoning array of bruises.

"What'll happen to Andrew now?" she asked.

I shrugged. "Not my department. After about his tenth DWI, and driving after revocation of his license, he may have to face a consequence this time."

I wrote orders for her release from the hospital. "I want to see you in the office tomorrow," I said. "And try to get Andy to come, too." I turned to the door.

"Doc, wait." Marijoan gulped and struggled to draw a deep breath.

Puzzled, I returned to her bedside. She flicked her eyes: looked at me, at a corner of the room, out the window beside her bed. "Doc, see ... Andrew wasn't driving when all this happened."

I waggled a forefinger at her. "Do you want me to repeat lecture number seventeen about enabling? Taking the blame for his actions comes under that heading."

"No, Doc, I really was driving, and in fact ... well, see, he wasn't actually in the car with me."

"Not in—But Deputy Perkins said he was lying on the pavement, where he'd been thrown free of—What are you saying?"

She sighed, and her fingers twisted. "I'd been at work, was on my way home. You know how dark it is this time of year and I almost didn't see . . . something was lying in the middle of the road. I realized it was a person and slammed on the brakes. I jerked the steering wheel to the right and plowed into that deep ditch. I managed to get the door open and crawled through snow onto the road to see what it. . . . Doc, it was Andrew, passed-out drunk, half frozen besides." She covered her face with bandaged hands and shook her head, that same slow metronome of anguish.

"I was pissed, Doc, steaming. There he lays, our new car's smashed up, I feel like a punching bag, and blood's dripping from my face and arms, while him—like so many of the disasters he causes—he's lying there peaceful as a hound pup. He's so big and I'm only half his size. When I tried to drag him away, he started swinging at me, awkward, but it stung. After all these years of ups and downs—Will he be drunk tonight? Or will I find him sitting quietly watching the Twins on TV?— love takes a beating from that kind of uncertainty. I'd reached the point. . . . I'd dreamed about what it would be like if he died or killed himself one of those times. What crossed my mind right then, Doc. . . ." She yanked tissues from the little bedside box. "If I hadn't seen him in time, or if someone else had come along 'stead of me. . . ."

She honked into a wad of tissues. I dragged a chair beside the bed. "You're one classy lady," I said.

"Classy! I just confessed to being a monster."

"What I heard was honesty of the rarest kind." I stroked my chin. "That battered-up love you talked about: is there still life in it?"

She sighed like Atlas on a hard day. "He's the father of our kids. He works, even when he shouldn't 'cause of beer. Even when he's drunk he never takes after me, and he always vows he won't never again. I think he means it when he's saying it."

"Was that a yes?"

"God help me, yeah."

"Good. Then shall we make use of the opportunity fate has given us?"

"What *are* you talking about?"

"If Foghorn doesn't quit drinking, he's going to die, one way or another. Treatment at a hospital equipped to give him his chance is available."

"He won't go."

"Of course not, unless someone helps him get there. That's where you and I can become a . . . a pair of pliers."

"What?"

"Half of a pair of pliers—you alone, or me—is a nearly worthless tool. No grip, no leverage. Put the halves together—both of us—and we can grip a problem even as tough as Foghorn. You'd have to not back down, though."

"Couldn't the sheriff just arrest him?"

"I don't know if lying drunk in the middle of a public road is illegal. If *he* had been driving, now. . . ." I peered at her over the top of my glasses.

She nibbled a fingernail. "If he *had* been driving . . . what?"

"That business of DWI and no license: I'm pretty sure that's a no-no."

She sampled a different nail. As the saying goes, a look of wild surmise crossed her face. She nodded abruptly. "If I really do love Andrew. . . ."

I nodded briskly.

"If we don't do something, he's going to die?"

More vigorous nodding.

"So." She inspected her ruined nails, then glanced at me. "Doc, I might of lied before there. Actually, Andrew was driving, and, uh, he was . . . weaving all over the road, and when we got to . . . I might of told him to be careful, and he might of jerked the wheel when he turned to tell me to mind my own business, and we might of gone into the ditch, and he might of gone flying out the door onto the pavement. Yep."

I beamed. "That being the case, we might enlist Deputy Perkins and petition Judge Maxheiner to issue an order putting him into treatment. He needs to spend weeks, not days, in the state hospital. A court order lets it happen. At the same time, you can work on your particular alcohol-related problem."

"My—I don't drink!"

"Enabling is part of the family aspect of alcoholism. You can learn how to not protect Foghorn from the consequences of his behavior—"

"Doc!"

"—instead of covering up for him. 'Taint easy, Marijoan, but it's learnable. Living sober's worth some effort."

"He'll fight like an Irishman."

"I happen to know that Les'd take kindly to seeing your husband in treatment instead of in jail."

Her lips drew tight. "I ain't usually one to lie, 'specially to a judge."

I scratched my chin again. "Person needs to define lying. Ever tell your kids there was a Santa Claus?"

She sat straight up in bed and skewered me with a blue-eyed Norwegian stare. Then I detected the ghost of a grin.

"Why, Doc!"

There came a knock on her hospital door, and Deputy Perkins called, "Can I come in?"

Marijoan Johannsen said, "We were waiting for you, Les."

He said, "I just need someone to give me a lucid story as to what happened last night. Foghorn's so blacked out he can't remember squat."

She lay back on her pillow. "What happened, Les ... see, Andrew picked me up from work. He'd been drinking again, scared me half to death, the way he was driving. When the car spun into the ditch, he went a-flying out onto the pavement. Doc and me, we been thinking that it was time for Andrew to get some help."

I went to the door of her room, shielded a thumbs-up from Les, and winked.

Thanks to the courage of a classy lady who cared enough to abandon enabling, my friend Foghorn confronted his alcoholism and "went into treatment." It wasn't easy, but then it never is. He worked his way through feelings of betrayal (anger), denial ("Who says I'm a drunk?"), and recognition ("I'm a worthless shit."), emerging into the warm sunshine of acceptance ("I'm not unique, and my family accepts me!"). A couple who has been through the pepper mill of "treatment" acquires a special glow: strength from admission of powerlessness; closeness between two who have found independence. Life.

The Vet Is In

VETERINARIANS were even scarcer than MDs in the far north. During the early years of my practice, I was occasionally called on to treat animals.

The Ekmans once asked me to stop by their farm and take a look at a horse. Darndest thing I ever saw: puffy all over, clear to the tips of its ears, as though it had been blown up with a pneumatic hose. Seemed to be edema, water trapped in the tissues. In people medicine, there is a condition known as anasarca—profound generalized edema—arising from an underactive thyroid. I wondered if horses ever grew goiters. Need to ask a real vet.

I ogled the beast.

"What is it, Doc?" Ron Ekman asked.

"It's all puffy," I said solemnly.

"That's it? Your diagnosis?"

"Yep."

"What should I do?"

"Darned if I know."

.   .   .

Gust brought his spaniel to the office one day. Frisky had had the poor judgment to challenge a dog twice his size, and a long gash ran from his shoulder along one flank.

"I have some ketamine we can use to put him to sleep," I said.

Gust said, "I don't like that idea. Frisky is my best friend. He'll understand. I'll just hold him."

"I don't know, Gust."

"Go ahead, Doc."

"Well—"

At the first prick of a Novocain needle, gentle Frisky turned into Stephen King's Cujo. It took five minutes to stitch up Frisky after I zonked him with the anesthetic. Then I spent an hour sewing up all the gashes in Gust's chin.

.   .   .

Agnes J. brought her "darlin'," a scrawny Boston bulldog named Bear Bait, to the office. Wheezing from an asthma attack, he sounded like a frantic teakettle. I've forgotten what impulse led me to order a chest x-ray, but I do recall deciding doggy lungs didn't look *that* much different from people lungs.

Beginning in the 1960s, a fine radiologist named Gib Wheeler interpreted all of our x-rays during a once-a-week visit to Northpine. I had forgotten that Bear Bait's film was among those waiting to be read.

It is so easy to become a captive of routine. To one scanning a stack of x-rays, an image of a small chest means it is that of a child. It took Gib a moment of confusion to realize that the film in hand was not a humanoid with a subtle miscue of nature but rather a ringer. I'm not sure he ever believed I didn't purposely try to fool him. I mean, if our roles had been reversed, that mischievous radiologist would have thought it great fun.

.   .   .

My ultimate veterinarian exploit still brings a blush to my cheeks. Barbara and I had acquired a female beagle puppy in the mistaken belief that our kids should have the experience and accompanying discipline of caring for a pet.

Ha!

We named her Lady. She turned out to have the intelligence of a grasshopper. Then arose the business of "going into heat."

It happened that the local high school math teacher had once entertained the idea of attending medical school. He later thought better of such an ill-advised notion, but as preparation he had hired on as an assistant in the medical school physiology department. Dog lab: where prospective surgeons test nascent skills with a scalpel. Well, they have to learn somewhere. Dick's job was to help sew the dogs back together. Of course, as a future general practitioner, I had not been invited near the place. To say that my personal acquaintance with doggy-innard anatomy was sketchy understates the matter by a country mile.

One evening Dick and I fell to discussing the issue of incipient canine fertility and the dearth of veterinarians available to interfere with it.

Dick said, "RAM, I'll help if you operate."

Me? People are one thing, but a dog?

Tempus fugits, and Lady developed an interest in roving, so one evening Dick and I set up in the treatment room. I achieved anesthesia with ether, turned that task over to Barbara, and Dick and I opened up Lady's tummy.

That's when the confusion arose. A dog's internal anatomy, while not radically different from a person's, doesn't look *exactly* the same. I prepared to remove the ovaries, but Dick said, "I think those are the kidneys."

"Ovaries," I said firmly. "They snuggle up to the Fallopian tubes."

"Kidneys," Dick insisted. "Who's the one who worked in dog lab?"

We debated until Barbara tartly suggested we get on with it.

We compromised. That's why Lady was the only hound dog in the whole county to have her tubes tied. Any breed, for that matter. Maybe in all of Minnesota!

Gol—ly.

Epidemic

A MOUNTAIN-CLIMBING ACQUAINTANCE of mine once was trapped partway up Mount McKinley in a storm, during which a series of avalanches cascaded through his camp, repeatedly burying his comrades and him under three to four feet of snow. He remembers most the feeling of absolute helplessness to avoid forces so out of his control.

Similarly out of one's control is the inevitable epidemic spread of some virulent infectious diseases. How does one avoid becoming the next victim? With diseases like poliomyelitis, before dependable vaccines hobbled it, there was no clear situation to avoid that would keep one safe. At least a disease like modern-day AIDS, as devastating as it is, leaves an understandable trail from victim to victim.

Half a dozen of Northpine's founding fathers were still alive when I arrived in town. One of these was Willie Willman, a patriarch among patriarchs. His Honor had been mayor for so long that folks could hardly remember whom he had replaced in the beginning. Once in a while some Johnny-come-lately thought about running against him, but residents quickly conveyed the error of such aspirations. In a town as small as Northpine, where members of better than half the populace were related to each other, differences of opinion easily escalated into regular Hatfield-and-McCoy affairs. To retain uncontested office for more than twenty years better described Willie's character than any breathless testimony.

Willie was a long-retired lumberjack, a title he wore proudly. He was shrewd and unflappable, a trait that kept a man alive as he rode a spring drive of thundering, pounding logs on some swollen northern river. And his blue eyes twinkled. Really.

Willie was born in 1878, which meant he was seventy-nine that epidemic year. I'd see him on the street regularly, we'd chat for a minute, and I'd depart his company brightened in a mysterious way.

December 1957 arrived with north-country briskness. In my Northpine office one morning, a pair of medical charts protruded from the rack beside Room Three. I looked at the labels: a matched set, Shorty and Mary, husband and wife.

After one glance at my patients, I dispensed with any cheery verbal fluff. "My God, did you two get run over by a steamroller?"

Doctors have a term for generic misery: general malaise—a wimpy phrase for what my friends radiated as they slouched on examination-room chairs. Eyes streaming, noses Rudolph-red and chapped, coughs savaging bronchial tubes already sandpaper raw, fever in the 104 neighborhood: Mary and Shorty barely acknowledged my presence.

"What's going on?" I asked.

Shorty muttered, "Went to Minneapolis. Brother's house. Everyone sick. Flu, I think."

Ah.

My first afternoon patient was Willie Willman. I hardly recognized the man as he slumped on my office chair, eyes closed. His temperature topped 104, his pulse was a snare-drum roll, his respirations were an obviously painful thirty-eight per minute. His chest was filled with wheezes and rales, sounds made by air bubbling past fluid seeping into the bronchial tree. The same bug that had claimed Shorty and Mary had a terrifying grip on our Mayor Willie.

I admitted him and started IV fluids and antibiotics. I gave him a dose of gamma globulin on the theory that desperately ill people were the ones on whom to use desperate measures. Gamma globulin is a concentrated fraction of blood serum containing some of the body's acquired weapons against bacteria and viruses, but its use is a shotgun approach to illness. Specific antibodies against the latest flu strain come only through exposure and conquest of the virus by a patient who survives the illness—too late to help an acutely ill person.

The state department of health sends notices when some new strain of the sneaky family of influenza viruses makes an appearance. This helpful hint is often a bit like tripping railroad-crossing flashers just after the train has run you over: tardy. Developing a vaccine based on that same new strain of the virus can yield results as timely as would be transportation provided to residents of Pompeii the day after. Whoever is in charge of such things named the 1957 strain of influenza "Asian Flu."

I called on Willie Willman several times a day. He developed pneumonia and a probable sinus infection, each a secondary bacterial infection. I broadened the scope of his antibiotics. His breathing became more labored, and his arterial oxygen content dwindled despite a heavy flow of the gas through a facial mask. He hung on.

. . .

The thing about a serious flu epidemic is that everybody, and I mean *everybody*, gets sick at the same time. If the virus is a pussycat strain, showing a few claws only when provoked, we all whimper and plow ahead. When the virus transmogrifies into a saber-toothed feline, call it Asian Flu.

Even the pussycat varieties are stealthy killers. Thirty-six thousand deaths occur from the disease in America during a typical year. In December 1957 and on through the winter of 1958, Father Death reaped a bonanza harvest. Picture an office-load of one hundred patients a day—made up of those who weren't too sick to wait around and be seen. Our twenty-bed hospital played host to forty patients, the nurses and doctors as miserable as all those patients expecting some elusive medical miracle.

On the fourth day I could not rouse Willie. His labored breathing was audible clear out to the nurses' station. He had no blood kin that anyone knew of, but the waiting room saw a flood of friends, "family" if you will, waiting, waiting, waiting.

I made a house call to the hamlet of Orr—sixty-three miles away—during the height of the epidemic. I vaguely recall examining a gaggle of people at the Johnson home, but because of my own delirium and spectacular fever I have no recollection of my trip back to Northpine. I must have made it because I answered the telephone in our bedroom when it rang at 3:00 AM. I dragged to the hospital, there to find a patient nearly as sick as I.

I was at his bedside on that fifth day when Willie Willman drew his last breath. I'm convinced he would have counted his life a good one, and I can nearly hear his voice assuring me of the fact. Still, dang it, the Willie Willmans of this world are rare enough that one could hope a benign Nature might look the other way when one such as he stumbles.

Doctors have an axiom about who will be most seriously affected by flu: the very young, the very old, the very ill, and the very pregnant. We lost half a dozen Northpiners, all from that "very old" contingent. Secondary infections—pneumonias, ear and sinus infections—lurk opportunistically, but toxicity from the virus itself can kill, and flu is not responsive to penicillin.

As I reflect on my forty-six years of active practice, I can claim that month at the beginning of the Asian Flu epidemic as the most trying of my career. I can only imagine what the flu pandemic of 1917–18 must have been like. When it comes to playing chess with Mother Nature, a colleague, Dr. R. E. Losee, put it well: "Keeps you humble."

Acute Stoppage of the Heart

U NDER OLD ENGLISH LAW, a coroner is charged with determining a cause of death in accidents, homicides, and
suicides. "Body found" cases, those people who have died while
not under a physician's care, represent a bit more of a challenge,
if accurate diagnosis is desired.

First elected county coroner on November 2, 1954, I served
for a total of twenty-four years. For the previous two decades, a
non-medical fellow had held the office, largely because few
seemed to care that in 90 percent of cases "acute stoppage of
the heart" was his official cause of death. Of course, in a way
he was right: stoppage of the heart and death do coincide with
remarkable regularity. Regarding my qualifications, as an avid
mystery reader I may have been particularly suited to the work,
at least that's what my brother-in-law thought. In honesty,
nothing in the medical school curriculum had uniquely prepared me to be a coroner. Circumstances taught along the way.

People assume that as a coroner I was regularly immersed
in Perry Mason—like mysteries. Truth to tell, unattended
deaths, the most frequent kind with which I was involved, were
usually pretty obvious and mundane. Even cases in which party
A did in party B, there was seldom any uncertainty as to why A
acted as he or she did, or as to whom A and B were.

A sampler of cases is a somber book of the dead: despair, virulent hatred, the pounce of stroke or heart attack, the consequence of a careless moment.

.   .   .

In only one instance, out of the hundreds of cases I supervised, was there a situation even remotely mysterious. The call came at 2:30 AM one Saturday. Typical: folks who drive off the highway plastered to the gills or who wait until closing at the friendly neighborhood tavern before deciding to shoot each other tend to need a coroner in the middle of the night.

Margery Jankowski was a widow, a white-haired wisp almost as skinny when viewed from the front as from the side. She lived alone in a small house out beside huge Lake Koochiching, some thirty miles from Northpine. She had a son who lived a few miles away, but she was something of a loner otherwise. People were accustomed to not seeing her about.

At about nine one Friday evening, Margery's son Phil tried to call her on the phone and, concerned at not reaching her, went to her cabin. He found lights on and the front and back doors locked. Peeking through a window, he spied Margery lying on her bed. When his banging and hollering brought no response, he broke the latch on the front door. His mother was obviously dead, so he called the local undertaker, who arrived about 11:30 PM and hauled Margery's body to his mortuary.

Right there is where the mortician, call him Alvin, went astray, because when a body shows up unexpectedly the coroner and the sheriff are supposed to be notified before anything else is done. The way Alvin explained it to me was that he "hated to call so late at night, you being clear down in Northpine and all."

As is usual practice, he removed her clothing, only to discover a neat little bullet hole in the notch just below her ribs.

Deputy sheriff Roger Edwards and I assembled at Alvin's mortuary to confirm that Margery indeed had the wound he described. The hole through her nightgown was surrounded by a halo of burnt gunpowder, proof that the weapon had been held against her when it was fired. We rounded up Phil Jankowski and returned to Margery's cabin.

No weapon was in evidence. All the windows and doors had been securely fastened until Phil had broken in. We had a genuine locked-door mystery.

Deputy Edwards and I searched the cabin. He did his things with fingerprint dust, finding only prints that we subsequently traced to Margery herself. He fiddled with locks and windows, concluding that they were too simple, too effective, to have been manipulated from outside. A little blood stained the bed, apparently a discharge from the rectum, no more than an ounce or two.

Dawn found us still prowling about the place. By this time, Rog and Phil were on hands and knees, scouring grass and brush around her house. With nothing else left unsearched, I started through drawers in a corner chest, some twenty feet from the bed where Margery had lain. In the bottom drawer, under slips and the kind of underwear little old ladies favor, I found a long-barreled .22 pistol. Smudged prints seemed to be hers.

That afternoon, Deputy Edwards, the county attorney, and I sat in the courthouse to sort out our confusion. Our conclusion, in the absence of evidence to the contrary: Margery had shot herself once in the abdomen, had gotten up and tidily placed the weapon in its hiding place, and then had crawled back in bed to await death. An autopsy revealed that the pellet had lodged in her spine without injuring the cord. It had punctured her small bowel and nicked the aorta, causing her to bleed to death internally.

The following Monday, in belated confirmation, her attorney received a suicide note in the mail. Margery had decided life was no longer worthwhile.

.   .   .

Your average Scandinavian is as laconic as a clam with lockjaw, relying on a head nod if even "Amen" is too wordy. Such reticence can lead to complications. With a wee apology to my Norwegian friends and relatives, I relate this true story, one involving a colleague.

Mrs. Yontson calls him one night at 3:00 AM. "Doc, my husband died," she says.

"Really? I'm sorry."

"Ja, dose t'ings happen."

"Well. If there is anything I can do—"

"I yust tau't you should know."

"Yes. Thanks."

Mrs. Yontson now calls Jim, the undertaker. "My Olaf, he's gone."

Jim, two-thirds asleep, says, "Where did he go, Mrs. Yontson?"

"To heaven. Maybe."

"You mean he's dead?"

"Dat's it."

"Have you called the doctor?"

"Ja."

"All right. I'll be there in half an hour."

At the mortuary, Jim and his helper lift Olaf's body onto the prep table and pull on rubber work gloves. Jim hears a prolonged groan.

"Somethin' the matter, Carl?" Jim asks his helper.

"Not with—"

The body on their prep table raises its arms, stretches, and sits up. Jim acknowledges later that he had never before fainted. He takes Olaf home, this time in the front seat of the hearse, and jumps all over poor Mrs. Yontson: "You told me you called the doctor to come and see Olaf!"

"No, I call, tell him Olaf is dead. You know, dat man always been a deep sleeper."

. . .

Zeke Johnson worked in the woods. As was still customary in 1955, his employer, Randy Fastern, supplied half a dozen crude shacks on skids as sleeping quarters for his men. Shaped like boxcars, made of splintery old boards, furnished with flophouse accessories, they were designed for men whose tastes were impossible to offend.

Snow began falling lightly just as the crew put away tools and trudged off for the night, each man to his own few cubic feet of shelter. The snow continued until morning, laying down a patina of fluffy whiteness. At dawn, "the boys" assembled beside Randy's office shack for instructions. They were in the bleary-eyed state of men who court sleep with half a pint of gin. Randy counted noses. "Where's Zeke?"

Big Ole looked around. "He ain't here."

"I know he—Holden, go bang on the door of his shack."

Holden shambled down the line of wooden cartons, pounded as instructed, pushed open the door, peered inside. He jumped back as though bee-bit—this according to Big Ole—and ran to the others like a lamed steer, gasping, "I t'ink he's dead."

I arrived at Randy's camp an hour and fifty miles later. A mishmash of gawkers' footprints had compacted the snow before Zeke's door. All insisted, though, that no footprints had come near Zeke's shack until Holden made his discovery. Deputy sheriff Tom Ejerdahl arrived, and we entered the tiny room together.

Randy's records indicated that Zeke was fifty-nine years old. The man wore the same pitchstained, ragged clothes he had finished work in the night before. His body sprawled across the cot, his feet on the floor, his trunk at right angles to the bed, his hands open-palmed at his sides. He was cold and very dead. Rigor mortis was full. Another of those "body discovered" situations, a typical coroner case. Except…

A long-barreled .22 revolver lay on the floor, five feet in front of him. Both Big Ole and Rat Root Swanson swore that it was Zeke's. Sheriff Ejerdahl picked it up gingerly. "Fired recently. One empty shell."

So now "body discovered" was transmogrifying into "probable suicide by gunshot." True, there was no final declaration of despair, but lumbermen were not given to angst-filled odes. Murder seemed ruled out by the blessing of pristine snow, devoid of tracks. Except…

We found no bullet wound.

We moved Zeke's body to Northpine, where the sheriff and I stripped it, checking, checking, checking.

"Okay, Doc Coroner," Tom Ejerdahl said, "tell me how a man can shoot himself dead and not leave a bullet hole. From what we found, I visualize him sitting on the edge of his bed, holding the gun at arm's length before him, pulling the trigger with his thumb. I found no pellet or bullet hole in the shack, and you can see none in him or his clothing."

Doctors are often accused of resorting to batteries of tests when they haven't a clue as to what is going on. I didn't know how to answer Tom, so I ordered x-rays.

Those of Zeke's head showed a .22 slug in the center of his skull. Thus primed, I used a light and speculum to determine that a slight blackening of his nasal turbinates was significant. By weird chance, with a pistol fired at arm's length, the bullet had entered Zeke's head precisely through one nostril.

. . .

A trip along Lake Superior's rocky shores provides vistas reproduced in many a photograph album. Two couples, friends riding in separate cars—the husbands in the one behind, their wives in the lead—headed toward Northpine. The women's vehicle careened off a highway curve and crashed down a boulder-strewn slope, exploding into flame. A car fire augmented by its own fuel burns with a crematorium's fury, and, there being no fire-extinguishing equipment within thirty miles, the flames had their way. The men and a growing crowd of other motorists watched helplessly.

While it takes a surprising amount of heat to consume a torso, extremities are more quickly reduced to minute fragments of bone. Such was the case here.

A wrecker brought the burned-out hulk to town and parked it behind Stu's Chevrolet garage, where I caught up with it. The car's floor was littered with tiny bits of debris that included what was left of arms, legs, hands, and feet. I donned a face mask and was probing through this material, looking for I knew not what, when a hand on my shoulder jerked me backward.

"What are you doing?" a florid-faced masculine stranger demanded.

My explanation did nothing to erase a scowl of suspicion from the man's face. "I want you out of there!" he snarled.

"Who—?" I began.

"Her husband. What did you find?"

"Oh, sir, I'm sorry. This must have been a terrible—"

"Show me!"

"Having to watch this happen and not be able to—"

"I demand to know what you took out of there!"

"Took out? Tiny fragments of bone are all that re—"

He pushed me aside and leaned into the space beneath the

melted steering wheel. "If I don't find it, you're going to hear from me!"

It was my turn to yank him out of the way. "It? It? What the hell are you—"

"Her diamond ring! It's worth—" He named a figure miles out of my price range.

I left him pawing through the detritus of his wife's existence.

· · ·

Empathy: the intellectual identification with or vicarious experiencing of feelings, thoughts, or attitudes of another, according to *Webster's Unabridged Dictionary*.

By this definition, I have a well-developed bump of empathy. A gift or a curse? Depends. My empathetic imaginings particularly awoke when I was called to the scene of a suicide. What manner of despair leads L. R. to drive from Minneapolis to a remote lookout cliff near Northpine and hang himself from the branch of a cedar tree? Or what impels K. K. to register in a local motel before blowing off his head with a large revolver?

In the case of woods worker Eric Brenderson, I at least believe I understand.

Jason Townsend was one of Eric's drinking buddies. One Saturday night, on the way home from an evening at Fuhrsen's Tavern, Eric lost control of his ancient GM truck. When it ceased rolling end over teakettle, Jason lay dead along the highway and Eric had sustained a broken arm. I reduced Eric's fractures and placed his arm in a cast. Jason, of course, entered county records as the latest coroner case.

Eric returned for scheduled follow-up care. I changed his cast at three weeks, providing one with a snugger fit.

Then Hoven, a fellow woods worker, found Eric in the tiny

cabin the man called home. He was dead, his head split from the violence of a .30-06 hunting rifle, its muzzle held in his mouth. A grisly wound, but far from unique. Except...

There were bloody handprints all over Eric's cabin. A basin of bloody water, several towels soaked red, smear marks from someone's attempt to clean up. Deputy sheriff Dick Ellison investigated the site with me. Two shells had been fired; two bullet holes had pierced the shack's thin walls. The bloody palm prints had been made by Eric himself.

Our reconstruction?

A suicide sometimes responds to a last-second preservation reflex. The firearm jerks in that desperate fragment of time, and the bullet fails to kill, what is termed a hesitation shot. For Eric, it must certainly have hit him somewhere in the face.

I am drawn unwillingly into his mind: guilt over his friend's death, a decision to atone, agony from the hesitation shot, resolve no longer as secure. Pump a basin of water, crawl about sponging up blood, throw aside the rags, return to the rifle, hold its stock between his feet, stare into its forgiving muzzle, grope for a trigger slippery with blood.

There are times when empathy is a doctor's best asset. There are times when it keeps him awake nights.

Seymore Adams

THERE WAS A TIME in the early sixties when medical opinion favored keeping a heart attack patient in the hospital for three to four weeks. I hesitate to call the idea a fad. Still, with medicine, as with so many practices, some things work better than others and outcomes can be hard to predict. For generations, heart attacks, if recognized at all, had been dealt with rather cavalierly—return to plowing the south forty as soon as the pain subsided, for example—leading to quite a few disasters. In belated recognition that a heart needed more time to heal, for a while we went overboard with hospital stays. Of course, back then the cost of a room in our ICU was about twenty dollars a day, so at least we weren't operating on some guy's wallet.

Northpine being a tourist attraction, three-fourths of our heart attack patients came from exotic places like Miami, Los Angeles, Des Moines, Omaha, and the Twin Cities. As a consequence of a prolonged hospital stay, Mr. Cardiac Case and I often got to be pretty good friends. Relationships became congenial, relaxed. Usually.

I recall an exception: Pete from Pittsburgh. Pete's attack was on the near side of major, but after a couple days his type-A-plus personality reasserted itself. He stormed out of the hospital over my strongly voiced dissent and headed home. He made it; a letter filled with brusque assessments of my character and ancestors verified the fact.

Then there was Seymore Adams.

Seymore chose Northpine as the place to have his heart attack. During the first while after such an event, a doctor is busy with details like keeping the patient alive, paying little attention to names or demographics. With Seymore, I spent the wee hours of the first night becoming well acquainted with his heart and lungs, taming erratic rhythm, propping up blood pressure, easing pain, squeezing any build-up of fluid out through his urinary catheter. It wasn't until the next day that someone discovered who our latest patient was and let me know.

Seymore Adams was a really, *really* VIP in a fraternal organization known familiarly as the Mafia. He called Chicago home; I elected not to ask what he was doing so far afield. Probably none of my business anyway.

The morning after his admission, I stepped into Room Two, our ICU. Comfortable; oxygen flowing; color pink; blood pressure 125 over 78; pulse regular at 88—these were the patient's vitals, of course. My pressure? Rising. Respiratory rate: increased. Pulse: sort of galloping. I recall wondering how his brethren might regard a less-than-topnotch outcome. Such speculation might have been a factor in *my* vital signs.

A pair of stolid, hulking men sat next to Seymore's bed, one on either side. When I cocked an inquiring eyebrow at the nearest, he rumbled, "Brother-in-law." The other just looked; him—to myself—I came to regard as Scarface. When I suggested that they might want to leave the room, they declined.

I could live with that.

The next three weeks were considerably longer than most

periods of the same duration. I'm not sure if Einstein ever explained that aspect of time's elasticity. Scarface and Brother-in-Law were present every time I made rounds. Maybe they knew how to sleep sitting up, eyes open. They never interfered with what I had to do; they just watched. Closely.

The day came when Seymore was ready to be discharged. He paid for his stay in cash. Before he marched out between Brother-in-Law and Scarface, he solemnly handed me a fishing rod and reel, by far the most expensive sports equipment I have ever owned.

I waved good-by from the back entrance of the hospital, and then relaxed so completely that I stumbled over the little metal threshold.

I'm grateful that things turned out well. Still, it would have been nice if they had smiled at least once. I suppose success in their line of work doesn't depend on bonhomie.

The Elephant in the Living Room

I INHERITED JANICE LLEWELLYN from another physician who had moved away from our area. She was the wife of a locally prominent businessman, a pillar in civic affairs, a nice person. She introduced herself that day in my office with a request for her "regular" refill of the tranquilizer Valium.

"How many have you been getting?" I asked.

"A hundred at a time."

"And for how long?"

"Goodness, Doctor, I can't remember. Years."

"Your usual dosage is?"

"The little yellow ones. Four a day, never more."

I thought, here we go again, and sighed. "Mrs. Llewellyn, do you realize that these have the potential to cause habituation?"

"Oh, I never use more than were prescribed."

"Four a day, a total of twenty milligrams, over extended time, is more than enough to set up ongoing need."

"I don't *need* them, Doctor."

"Good. We'll taper you off and—"

"Wait, now. I won't be able to sleep if you do that!"

"I am ethically opposed to contributing to dependency on a drug. I'll see you through the withdrawal period so that you—"

"Doctor, I've never heard such nonsense! I'm a devout Christian and would never consider becoming 'dependent' on a drug!"

"I'm glad you feel that way. It will make it easier—"

"Besides, these are not *drugs!* They're medicine."

We discoursed for half an hour. I explained about a drug's "half-life," the time required for 50 percent of a given dose to be excreted from the body: twenty-four hours in the case of Valium; how after such prolonged use her body was saturated with the chemical, that it would take weeks before she was completely free of its effects. She went from surprise to indignation to roaring anger to pleading to sullen acceptance. I'm not sure why she didn't flounce out of the office in search of a more "understanding" physician.

Over the next weeks, I gradually weaned her off the drug. She insisted that during her first month of total abstinence she had not slept a single minute of the entire thirty days. I could only assume that she had flitted in and out of brief periods of exhausted sleep unawares.

The upshot? Six months later, Janice was off the medication and somehow, improbably, we had become friends. If only stopping chemical nirvana were as easy as starting.

. . .

I have never met anyone whose life goal was to become addicted to a drug. Nurse Sarah had put it poignantly: "Doc Rowland din't set out to get hooked on the sauce." That so many end up in those hazardous waters reveals the insidious nature of the process. Use of a chemical to solve a personal problem is so pervasive that we rarely regard it as aberrant. To many, alcohol is an essential lubricant to socializing. Need something for pain? Can't sleep? Nerves wound tight? Depressed? Are we not the Prozac generation? Ask your friendly physician and she or he will respond with a conditioned reflex: take pen to prescription pad. Sometimes this is not only harmless but a sort of kindness garbed in therapy. But when temporary surcease becomes agonizing need, when chemical dependency (CD) claims another victim, then indeed does an elephant, whose existence must be denied, take up residence in the living room.

· · ·

Convincing someone saddled with the medical problem of CD to acknowledge and do something about it is nearly always a challenge. The exceptions stand out like Lake Superior lighthouses during a November gale. Consider Old John, an example for the ages:

John's complaint was direct. "Doc, I'm a mess. Send me to Moose Lake." The state hospital there treated alcoholism.

I did.

John returned home in due time, inveigled use of a closet in the courthouse basement, and solemnly conducted weekly AA meetings, complete with readings from the AA Big Book, recitation of the famous serenity prayer, and meditation—entirely by himself.

Then something mysterious, even awesome, happened: Fremont joined him, and there were two. Jansen began coming, then Shirley and George, a married couple, and Trixie and Conrad and Jim . . . word spread about the healing occurring in that dark corner of hopelessness. Old John was literally the founder of Northpine's successful Alcoholics Anonymous and treatment aftercare response. Would that a more public acclaim could be awarded this humble giant of a man, but that "anonymous" injunction gets in the way. Still, many of us know, John, and we thank you for your courage.

· · ·

Sixty-two-year-old Abigail arrived at the Northpine Hospital one evening with complaints of chest pain and an odd tingling down her left arm. It was quickly apparent that she was having a myocardial infarction, a classical heart attack. Heart disease is not exclusively a guy thing.

I admitted her, worked her up, and used all the medical tricks then available to ameliorate the damage a plugged coronary artery creates. We settled in to become acquainted over the next few days.

Her husband looked vaguely familiar, allowing for worry lines and the fatigue of his bedside vigil. Then I put together a couple of twos. "You aren't—" I said his name, that of a Minneapolis TV personality.

He confessed that he was. "We love to get away to Northpine whenever we can, but this time Abigail—Well, you diagnosed it."

I was pleased to meet the icon in person and even more pleased that things were going so well. And they did. Until—

When I made rounds the third day, nurse Edna Freeman wore her anxious look.

Uh-oh.

Edna said, "It's Abigail. Ever since she woke up this morning, she's been—different. I believe she's hallucinating."

Hallucinations are not among the standard symptoms of a heart attack. I stood beside Abigail's bed and watched while she plucked invisible somethings out of the air. When I spoke, she paid me scant attention. Her husband sat in the corner, his face ashen. I gazed inquiringly at him. His sigh stretched the limits of a breath. "I should have told you. Abigail has a—God, this is so hard. She's a wonderful woman, has been a Good Housekeeping mother to our children. I think my job, the hours, the responsibilities—She drinks a pint of brandy every day. I didn't realize what would happen if she quit."

I was able to thwart full-blown delirium tremens by use of a more acceptable sedative than brandy. From that day on, I never failed to nail down a heart attack patient's extent of alcohol use.

So, even genuine ladies can become dependent on chemical crutches. I never heard, but I hope brushes with death twice in three days broke through Abigail's denial and that she learned how to live without brandy or its pharmaceutical equivalents.

· · ·

Consider Ted. His daughter and I sat beside his hospital bed, where he was again recovering from the ravages of a binge.

"I'm sending you to Duluth for alcoholism treatment," I said.

"No way. I'm not going."

"Yes, you are."

"No, I'm not."

"Yes, you are."

"The hell you say."

"Yes, you are."

"When am I going?"

Like that.

· · ·

A colleague, call him Doctor, hiding behind the delusion of denial, had come to the attention of the state medical society. The man was a friend—a talented, caring, energetic physician—and he was on the path toward family disintegration and professional disgrace due to his increasing dependence on alcohol. A state medical society official enlisted my help.

I spent a couple of sessions with Doctor. He steadfastly refused to consider hospitalization and treatment. Then one day, as I was driving home from a visit with an R-PAP medical student in a rural community, I happened to pass Doctor's town. On impulse, I swung off the freeway and went to his office, bullied my way past guardians at the front desk, and cornered him in the clinic library.

I ended my "final" plea that he accept CD treatment with, "If I had a magic button that would send you into the hospital, I would—" I pressed my finger on the table.

He regarded me solemnly. "When do you want me to go?"

"My car's out front."

I took him directly to the treatment facility. As they say in the jargon of the profession, he "got a good program" and became a leader in the fight to save dependent colleagues.

Thank God for magic buttons. Sometimes the elephant in the living room finally becomes visible.

Aristotle

MANY TIMES during my years of front-line practice along Minnesota's northern border, I met situations where laughter seemed the only alternative to tears. Case in point: Aristotle.

Aristotle Despopalous was from Detroit. This detail probably has nothing specific to do with the events I'm about to relate. He arrived in our county one morning at 3:10 AM, piloting an expensive convertible of some kind. Does Porsche make such a model? I'm not into cars. Suffice to say, it was a toy to gladden the heart of your average plutocrat.

The night was foggy, perhaps a factor in what happened. Our broad Highway to the Outside was a marvel of engineering: well-announced curves swept around cliffs, creating virtually no hazard to a driver.

The highway engineers did not reckon on Aristotle Despopalous.

A basic law of physics decrees that if Road A veers to the left, Automobile B would do well to follow suit. Despopalous flouted the law. Speed entered into the equation as well. We later came to realize that Aristotle never monitored such mundane devices as speedometers, instead occupying himself with Deep Thoughts.

His car flew off the edge of a curve, straight as a beam of light into the stygian gloom. Rattle, tumble, crash, slam: wreckage littered a swath chewed by the disintegrating car, which came to rest 132 feet away from highway macadam.

Aristotle crawled free of the most expensive pile of junk ever seen in these parts. He hitched a ride into town with Rob Kramer. Rob is Fritz's boy, the one who dates Liz Feebich down at—Well, that's another story. Thing is, he happened along because of his interest in Miss Feebich.

We convened at the hospital around 3:35 AM, I still one-quarter asleep but with eyes open, in the frame of mind I usually am at that hour: ready to stomp someone's foot. Aristotle lay stretched out on the emergency-room table. Well, sort of stretched out. Raised up on his elbows, actually, held in place by nurse Edna Freeman.

Rob said, "I saw this guy standing in the dang middle of the dang road. He was pointing toward town, jumping up and down like he was bee-bit."

I said, "Bees don't bite; they sting."

Rob said, "You want to hear this or not, Doc?"

"Sorry."

"This guy demanded to be taken to a telephone, said he had to call—I think he said, 'the Mater.' I got a good look at him, blood all down his side, only he didn't seem to notice. I says to him, 'What happened?' and he says, 'Flat tire.' I shined a light across the ditch—Doc, that car isn't decent scrap. I says, 'Man, you need a doctor,' and he says, 'I'll be the judge of that,' but I says—Doc, all the way to town he kept up the dangdest chatter about the dangdest things, about how he owns a bank, and he's a personal friend of President Eisenhower, and—unbelievable stuff."

I focused attention on Aristotle. About twenty-five, well dressed in a tattered and blood-splattered way, voluble. I found no injuries other than the obvious one, that to his forearm. The man had flensed it. A ten-by-three-inch patch of skin and subcutaneous tissues was missing. Muscles lay exposed in anatomy-book fidelity.

I asked if he had been knocked out.

"Heck no," Aristotle said. "I want a telephone."

"Sir, you have a remarkable wound."

"Slap on a bandage."

I said, "You don't understand. Too much is missing." Aristotle reared up and swung his feet off the cart. I grabbed his shoulder. "I have to cleanse the wound, dress it in preparation for skin grafting—"

"Is there a motel nearby?"

"—admit you for observation."

"Surely the motel would have a telephone."

"Antibiotics. Protective isolation. Sterile saline packs—"

Aristotle spied a telephone in the hallway and dragged us along behind him. He placed a collect call to Detroit. Whoever was on the other end refused to accept it.

By guile—okay, by outright deception—Nurse Freeman and I steered Aristotle to a bed in Room Two, where we wrapped his arm in sterile saline dressings. He beat us back to the nursing station, where he dropped the bandages in front of us.

"Icky, wet, sloppy," he said.

We corralled him again and bandaged his arm to resemble that of an Egyptian mummy. It took him nearly five minutes to remove the dressings. I explained in Firm but Simple Language, "Leave the *gol-ding-dong-dang* bandages alone!"

The next morning, halfway through office hours, nurse Jean Frances called to announce that Aristotle had vanished. Shortly thereafter, village police officer Louie Wagenknecht phoned from the Municipal Liquor Store and Lounge, where Aristotle was regaling the patrons, cadging drinks by showing his wound, wide open of course.

I plunked him down in his room and explained again about the dressings. "Keep your hands off those *blinking blanking blonking* bandages!" He grinned at me, and our simian ancestral ties had never seemed quite so evident.

I reached his mother by telephone. When I explained that Aristotle was our guest, she hung up. I called back. Mater Despopalous well hid any latent maternal feelings.

I said, "His behavior is ... different."

"He's crazy as a loon," she said.

Now, our beloved loons are stately, gorgeous creatures without a hint of erratic behavior. I drew breath to explain the discrepancy in her metaphor, but she hung up again. I called a third time, demanding to know what we should do with her boy. Hysteria lent timbre to my voice.

"Turn him loose. He always comes home."

"He no longer has a car!"

She mentioned airfare, Western Union.

I was unrestrained. "Oh, thank you, thank you, thank you. However, I don't consider him totally responsible. Who will come to escort him?" When she declined to volunteer and I said, "But he needs—" Mater Despopalous slammed down her phone.

We reserved a seat on a North Central Airline flight from Duluth to Detroit. Ray, our lab tech, agreed to deliver Aristotle to Duluth International Airport. A World War II veteran, Ray had seen duty in the south Pacific. The experience served him well as preparation.

He told it this way: "We sat in the back seat, I clamped onto his good arm the whole way. At the airport I got him as far as the gangplank when darned if he didn't take off at a gallop down the runway, hollering, "Vroom, vroom," flapping his arms, that bandage unwinding like a kite tail. The co-pilot and I rounded him up, and I headed for home."

No one ever came for the car. I've often wondered about Aristotle. Not enough to write, though.

In the Line of Duty

FOR TWENTY-FOUR YEARS I was a coroner, a part-time job in the sparsely settled north. Homicides, suicides, and "unattended" deaths comprise grist for a coroner's mill. The pay was a less-than-princely ten dollars per case, regardless of how much it chewed up my day, and the hours were predictably unpredictable—calls at 3:00 AM, or while tied up with an operation, or when the office was jammed, or when my kids were playing little league baseball, or during a tender moment with a long-suffering spouse.

Over the years I worked with many peace officers because the parameters defining my involvement naturally coincided with the responsibilities of sheriff or policeman. My respect for these men and women grew in proportion to my contact with them. I marvel that so many willingly serve the rest of us when low pay is the rule and acceptance by Joe Citizen is often snide if not actively hostile. Even in sylvan Northpine, an occasional thug is not above shooting at an officer.

Robert Peterson was a Minnesota State Highway Patrolman stationed in Northpine. Over the years he and I worked together on twelve or fifteen auto fatalities along the stretch of highway that was his beat, and even on one fatal stabbing for which he happened to be the closest policeman.

To say Bob and I were buddies squeezes the word a tad. We

respected each other. If our paths crossed, we would readily share a booth at Woody's Café for a Danish and coffee. To Bob, there were right ways and wrong, with little commerce between them; my eyes, on the other hand, seem tuned to an infinity of grays.

I have a talent for dressing in my Sunday best without destroying an aura of basic slobbishness—necktie mysteriously off center, shirttail breaking free, buttons awry. But Bob in uniform was a walking recruitment poster for the highway patrol: the brim of his hat a perfect plane, like maroon rings around a felt Saturn; the fabric of his jacket spotless, its sheen shellac, its buttons lined up parade-ground orderly.

Every man, however stoic, has a secret warm spot. Bob's was his daughter, his eyes expressive whenever he spoke of her.

I was at her bedside the night she died.

A doctor must report devastation: try to convince himself that it doesn't hurt, hope that his voice will see him through the task. My open mouth was mute when I went to the waiting room to find Bob. I threw my arms around that fierce warrior, and we sobbed together.

For several months my path did not cross Bob's. Then one day he stood beside his patrol car on Main Street, so I detoured and said, "Hey, Bob, how're you doing?'

He looked around in slow motion. "Oh, hi, Doc."

"Want a cup of coffee? On me."

He considered, staring across the street. "I don't have time right now. How about a cup of coffee instead?"

He saluted raggedly and crawled into his unit. A seam of his jacket had split, leaving a gap.

.   .   .

The days wore on. One afternoon nurse Elaine Andresen banged down the telephone and grabbed my arm as I went past her desk. "Out on the highway. Need you, RAM!"

I'm no Andretti, but when I have to I can wheel. I covered the thirty miles in a bit more than twenty minutes, dread bitter in my mouth, the scent of blood already in my nostrils. Once there, I clawed through a mushroom-ring of gawkers. Deputy sheriff Tom Ejerdahl was all but clubbing people back, directing traffic, snarling at lifelong friends, clearing the scene.

A van stood half off the pavement, its turn indicator blinking steadily. A car-length behind it sat a squad car, lights flashing with that whirly sound. Across the road were two other police vehicles.

Deputy sheriff Les Perkins knelt on the pavement amidst splatters of blood, pumping on the bared chest of a sturdy man sprawled on his back. Les spied me. "Oh God, Doc, am I doing it right? Should I be resusc—Bullet holes in his chest—Help me, Doc!"

I listened with my stethoscope to a chest that had fallen silent with suspension of the officer's efforts. Skin blue, lips purple, three holes in the front of the man's ribcage—such innocuous marks, pencil-sized, oozing but not gushing blood, just—enough. My curses and tears and inner storming didn't change it: Bob Peterson was dead. I shook my head at Perkins, who slammed a fist against the squad car door, denting steel as though it were tinfoil.

I found my voice. "Who—How did this—"

"Him!"

Les Perkins pointed past the hood of Bob's squad car, at the space between it and the still-blinking van, at the rag-doll body crumpled on itself, at a .22-gauge rifle and a policeman's .38

Smith & Wesson pistol lying nearby—all a dozen feet from where Bob lay.

I croaked, "Les, did you...?"

"No, Doc, this is what I found."

Officer Perkins ran to the side of the road, retching, his bloodstained uniform wet with sweat, now splashed with swamp water from the ditch. I steadied my knees by leaning against the hood of Bob's unit.

I yelled, "Someone turn off the damned squad-car lights!"

Deputy Tom Ejerdahl touched a switch, and then there was silence save for the van's blinker. I snarled, jerked open the van's door, and throttled it. I spun back to stand beside Bob.

Les and Tom measured and photographed, did those things officers must, no matter the victim. When the ambulance arrived, twenty willing hands lifted Bob tenderly onto its gurney. I returned to the other body, wondering, fighting cobwebs of confusion.

A woman wobbled out of the ring of spectators and lurched toward me and the officers where we clustered in silent bemusement. "He's been drinkin' all day," she mumbled.

"You know him?" I rasped.

"Hector, my husban'. He's been drinkin' all day."

"What happened!"

She looked up at me in slow motion, the way drunks do when they realize someone is speaking to them, eyes searching even though you are standing right there. "I was drivin' 'cause Heck coun' 'countta he was drinkin'—"

"Tell us," Les exploded.

"—an' I only had one drink. Or two. That officer come up behin' us with a si-reen screechin', so I pulled over an' he—he was lyin' righ' there—he banged on my win'ow and tol' me go back his car, only Heck said I din' need to, so that occifer—that man, started writin' a ticket, but he broke a pencil righ' two an' started back to that police car there, an' Hector, he grabbed our rat-killin' rifle an' jumped out the van, see. He ran aroun' behin'—I screamed an' yanked open my door, ran back there, too. The cop was standin' behin' the open door his car, reachin' for I s'pose a pencil, an'—But Heck, he, he shot at the policeman, righ' through the win'ow a that car, an' a, a red spot came on the cop's ches'—He straighten up an' yank that horrible pistol out, an', an' he pointed it right at Heck, so Heck had to shoot again a time or two, mebby, more holes through the win'ow tha' car a his, an' the cop he kep' aimin' right back, like in movies, an'—he had the oddes' look on his face before he sort of sat down an'—"

Her skittering eyes located Deputy Ejerdahl. "Do you got any Kleenex?"

"No. *Kleenex!* Is that when Bob shot that—your husband?"

She sniffled like a kid with a head cold. She seemed to consider, then shook her head. "The cop din' shoot Hector. He jus' kep' lookin' along that horrible gun a his, then his eyes sort of turned up an'—You sure you ain't got any Kleenex?" She snuffled.

Deputy Perkins snarled, "Get on with it!"

"When the cop fell down, his head banged on the pavemen' an' he dropped that gun a his. Hector ran over an' slap' his cheek, not hard, min' you. Like I seen onc't on *As the World Turns.*"

Les nearly grabbed the front of her jacket. "Then how did his service pistol get over there, and who shot that son of a—"

"Well, when the cop woun't say nothin', Heck, he screamed an', an' he turned his rifle 'round an' looked right into its barrel an' pulled the trigger, but it jus' clicked, woun't shoot. He ran over here an' kicked the van, righ' there, then back he went, grabbed that cop pistol an' held it in his mouth like you suck on a lollypop, him sorta runnin' backwards, an' he musta pulled the trigger."

If I had a time machine, I'd run it back to those five seconds, maybe ten, when Bob had Hector in his sights—aware, still on his feet, steadying his pistol atop the patrol-car door—to see for myself that look in his eye. Maybe then I would understand why he never fired his weapon.

Weird and Wondrous Wounds

R OLF SAID, "I was cutting brush when it felt like something
got into my eye, and it's been a little sore since."

Corneal abrasions and small foreign bodies stuck to the
transparent surface are common. I did my usual: anesthetic
drops to numb the touchy cornea, fluorescent dye and ultra-
violet lamp to highlight any abnormalities. Nothing.

"Gosh, Rolf, I don't see—"

Wait: a dark spot near the inner aspect of the orbit. I donned
magnifiers. It looked like a foreign body.

With tweezers I pulled out an inch-long thorn that had slid
in alongside the eyeball.

. . .

Sally Aagaard was the patient in Room Two of my Northpine
office. She held up her right hand, its middle finger showing the
typical flexion deformity of a so-called "baseball finger," the ter-
minal phalanx bent sharply toward her palm. The underlying
problem: the threadlike tendon fastened to the base of the last
finger bone on its dorsal side, that which allows a person to
fully straighten the finger, had torn free.

"Surely you haven't been playing softball in February,"
I said.

Sally sighed. "Nope. I work at the Best Western Motel, was
making up a bed, jammed my finger while I was tucking in a
sheet. Pretty stupid, huh?"

"No comment," I said. "Only, you're the third person I've treated for this injury from the same cause. I call it Bed-Maker's Lament."

. . .

Ellie had a sore foot, tenderness over the outer aspect at the base of her fifth metatarsal. X-rays confirmed presence of a fracture. It was not displaced, however, and would heal without prolonged trouble.

"How did this happen?" I asked.

"I sort of, like, fell."

"From much of a height?"

"No." I think she blushed. "Actually. . . ." She picked up her shoe, one of those fashion statements of a few years ago, its sole a couple of inches thick. "I fell off this darn thing."

. . .

Chick worked at a sawmill just outside of Northpine. One day the whirling blades of a planer dragged his hand through a slot intended for a one-inch plank. Time and a series of operations healed what was left well enough that my good buddy was able to grip a bowling ball and join a group of us seniors at the local lanes. Gratifying, except that, chewed-up hand and all, the son of a gun kept beating us.

. . .

The lad was eight. He waddled into my office one afternoon, ushered by his mother, Marie, who huddled over his whimpers and held a dishtowel around his waist.

I patted the end of my exam table. "Can you jump up here?" I asked.

He shook his head side to side urgently. I prepared to lift him.

"Careful, Doc," Marie said.

"Of what?"

"You wanna tell him?" she asked.

The boy shook his head again and swiped a tear from a cheek that was summertime grubby. I cocked an eyebrow at Marie and thought I detected the makings of a chuckle on her warm Irish features.

"Kids are always—He was playing with his brothers and—I don't know why kids always wait 'til the last second before they come in to—you'd think their bladder'd burst. After he did his job, he couldn't wait to get back out to—See, Doc, he zipped up before he was quite all tucked back inside and—"

So, how do you free a lad who has trapped a generous portion of his penis in the zipper of his trousers? Gently, sir, gently.

A Man Does ...

SOMETIMES THE MAJESTY of the human spirit reveals itself like a pearl, beauty layered about a piece of grit, hidden
away from casual view in the remote darkness of its parent
shell. I came to know Ole and his spirit when he cautiously laid
aside stoicism and shared of himself.

We sat beside the rickety table in Ole's "job" shack, his only
home. He winced and moved gingerly.

"The pain?" I asked.

Ole Olson clenched a hand gnarled by forty years spent in
logging and rubbed his belly. "That ache's been like a rat gnaw-
in', won't no longer obey friend whiskey. Last week you give 'er
a name, Doc. That carson—something—of the pan, pancr—
sweetbreads. You explained. I knew. Cancer's what you meant."

I could only nod.

Ole was lean and slight, tough like well-cured shoe leather,
a fifty-nine-year-old body made of muscle and gristle, skin
tough enough to dull a mosquito's probe. He was a logger who
remembered the days when chain saws were for sissies and a
horse snaked logs to the landing. Back then, men didn't quit;
they could do anything they set a mind to. Almost anything.

He shifted on his chair. "A man goes along without giving
death a thought. Sure, people die, even folks you knew. A tree
falls on a fellow, like Axel that time, but ... me?" He grinned sar-

donically. "I ain't never died, so I ain't never going to. You go to work or hang one on, have a fight as part of a drunk, chew the fat with the guys at Gordy's Tavern, visit a whore. A life. Only thing, it don't provide a man with anyone to much care. Not with family, or grandkids, no one like that little Jenny.

"Then comes a great swolled leech inside to suck out your juices and . . . and you're whipped, ate up alive. Death comes a-knockin', says, 'Howdy, Ole, you and me's going to get acquainted soon,' and I says back, 'Hell no, Mr. Death, I can keep ahead of you,' but that old man, he just grins at me there in the rearview mirror, him knowing, just waiting.

"Doc, when you told me all this a week ago, I figured Mr. Death was the enemy, but now that I've thought on it and found out what hurting can accomplish, now that I know I ain't *really* getting away, now that I see the other side of the ridge— maybe that old man . . . ain't so bad . . . as I thought."

Blinking back moisture, I stared out the open door of Ole's shack, at the hillside so recently shaved of trees, at the trailer of Ole's boss, Elmer Johnson, where he, Addie, and their little Jenny stayed, at the seven other shacks-on-skids lined up past Ole's, logging-camp homes for the crew. His was first in line because he was foreman, mayor of this Bachelorville.

"Wantta tell you, Doc," he said, "'bout last night. See, the pain gets worse as the sun goes down. Why is that?"

I shook my head. "I've heard that before. Maybe because that's the lonely time."

Ole nodded. "And then when ya run outta friend whiskey. . . . I sat there, holdin' the last empty bottle. No slosh left. Done, just like. . . ." He lumbered to his feet, stepped to the wall opposite the door, and lifted down a rifle from a pair of deer knuckles. He snapped it to his shoulder, sighted down its smooth, rust-free barrel, sniffed the comfort of gun oil next to his cheek, caressed the gleaming wood of its stock. He laid it on the table between us.

"Me and this lived together in the woods for fifty years," he said softly. "Never let me down. I'd decided.... Yesterday I asked it to do me one final favor. Sat in that chair, lined it up with the butt on the floor. 'Member wonderin' if I would see a foretaste of hell roar outta it just before.... Then's when Elmer Johnson stopped by. I quick-like slide the rifle under the table, try to act like ever'thing's okay. Elmer's as excited as that dang Swede knows how to get. 'Got the new contract,' he says, 'that sale over by the reservation. Need your help settin' up the new job; couldn't hardly do it without you,' he says."

Night had parceled out its minutes, and Ole counted every second. Daylight crept over distant spruce tree spires, but it brought no comfort. "Mr. Death," Ole muttered, "last night I gave you the finger, but today you look better'n ever. Things are getting nigh onto 'can't' when I think about setting up that new job." How could he get through the day, let alone a week? Why should he? screamed the pain. Did he owe anyone that much?

"That's when I run outta whiskey, Doc, with none closer than Northpine, thirty miles away. Gone, my friend, my only real friend."

Then he asked, "Have you met Jenny?"

I smiled. "I delivered her, have watched her grow."

His smile matched mine, and his eyes wanted to leak. I understood. Four years old, she was filled with candor and trust. Uncontaminated by the wiles of maturity, Jenny was a kind of purity, with hair as sunny as her nature.

Ole said, "She runs at me with arms outstretched, all the while a-screamin' my name. *She* is a friend. So, I hang in."

The afternoon sunbeams picked at the lock of dust and

grime on the shack's lone window. Ole hugged his belly and drew a shuddering breath. I reached into my doctor's bag and hauled out a bottle of morphine pills. "I can give you a shot," I said.

He considered, then shook his head. "Maybe later." From the table he picked up an ancient clock, ticking off life with mechanical fervor. "Last night I sat there, face to face with that monster. Figured a man should know the moment in which he dies." He touched the rifle. "It's a comfort to have nearby, Doc. Hope you understand."

I half closed my eyes, then nodded.

He laid the weapon across his knees, stroked it, glanced at me from the corner of his eye. I bit back any words. Then . . .

"Hi, Ole."

The rifle clattered to the floor. He gaped at the girl watching us solemnly from the square of sunlight she brought with her through the open door.

"Jenny, what—I—"

"Are you fixing your gun, Ole?"

His eyes glistened. "I'm—Ja, fixing . . ."

"You haf to be careful with guns. Daddy told me."

"Ja," he managed.

"I'm going away tomorrow," she said.

"Away?"

She twitched her nose in excitement. "Down to town." She kicked at a rough place on the floor. "You need to fix that, Ole, 'cause you might . . . if you trip . . . what if you got hurt?" Sunlight made her face glow with round-cheeked pinkness. Her blue eyes regarded Ole directly. "I'm going to Grandma's. I like to see her, but I'll be glad when I come back 'cause then we can talk some more. Bye."

She jumped to the ground, then looked back at Ole and smiled. "I love you," she called.

We watched her run, hair streaming, a golden flag waving at us. Her legs pounded all out as she strained toward the next moment in her life.

Ole picked up the rifle and caressed its sheen. He sighed and labored from his chair. My leg had gone numb, the muscles held so tight. Ole lent me a hand when I stood. He laid the gun on its deer knuckle holder, and we shook like two presidents sealing a pact.

"I'm glad to know you, Ole," I said.

He looked me square on. "Hell, Doc, a man does. . . ." The power of his grip told me what he meant. I stepped down to the ground and turned to give Ole a salute.

He knelt, studying the place in the floor that needed patching.

Miss Emerson

ONCE IN A WHILE NEIGHBORING COLLEAGUES covered another's practice so one of us could escape for a brief respite. For the patients of a relieved physician, there are pros (the New Broom Syndrome) and cons (this new doc doesn't understand a thing about me). For the stand-in doctor, it can be an adventure filled with new patients and new problems. I was on such a lark one summer.

Miss Minnie Emerson's chart was nearly two inches thick and had raggedy edges. I sighed as I hoisted it out of the rack beside Room One in Dr. Colleague's office. Doctors call a thick patient chart the Sears Sign. Nothing discourages thorough review of records more than a catalogue-sized patient folder crammed with data from a hundred visits.

Miss Emerson perched on the edge of her chair like a sparrow considering flight. She was wiry, had white hair, and hid any fatty tissue someplace out of view.

"Good morning, Miss Emerson, how are you to—"

"Come in, Doctor, have a chair, although these aren't very comfortable. Still, you supplied them. Well, perhaps not you specifically. You're new, aren't you?"

"Filling in for your physician, Dr. Colleague, while he takes a well-deserved—"

"Not *new* new, not with hair that color."

"Yes. What brings you here today?"

"I have a Ford."

"What? Oh, brings you—Uh, I meant, what is your problem to—"

"My father always said we were related to Ralph Waldo Emerson. Not on my mother's side of course."

"Your problem?"

"I don't have any problem. My father was so sure of it that he and Mother, at least I think she had a say in it, named my brother Waldo."

I tuned out and opened the chart, only to have pages scatter like goodies from a ruptured piñata.

"Oh my," she said, "things will be all mixed up. Let me help you."

We crawled around on hands and knees. I scooped up those sheets within reach and regained my chair.

"Miss Emerson—Please, you may sit again. Don't worry about those—Please?"

"When I was a girl, I was always spilling things, and do you know what my father did to cure me? He clapped his hands in front of my face."

"Like this?" I patty-caked politely.

"Oh my, no, not nearly vigorous enough."

I tried again. She beamed. "That sounded just like him."

"Good. Now, may we continue?"

"Where, dear?" she said.

"I need to know why you came in today."

"Because it was time. My father used to do that, clap his hands, and you reminded me of him right then, although you are much heavier, especially around the waist and under the chin, than he ever—"

I clapped again, with heart.

"Yes, dear?"

"Miss Emerson, I really need to know what it is time for, this visit today."

"Why didn't you say so? All you need to do is ask, I always say. I mean, how else can you—"

I clapped once more; I was getting into the rhythm. She laced her fingers across her lean little abdomen and regarded me expectantly. "Miss Emerson, how have you been feeling?"

"When?"

"Uh, recently."

"About the same."

"About the same as when?"

"Before."

"Which was?"

"It's probably in the chart. I can never remember when things happen, can you? Maybe I'm just getting old, that's what Birdie says, but she's worse than I am. Do you know, she—You look tired, dear. You people don't get enough sleep. When I was a girl, my father—"

"Stop! Uh, sorry. Look, for this interview to have any value—"

"What interview?"

"What I'm trying to—What I'm asking—Why you are *here*."

"Do you stutter, dear?" She clapped bony hands. "Father always said you could frighten a person out of—Oh no, that was hiccups."

I recall holding my head. She patted my shoulder. "Now you really look like Father, because he used to do that quite often."

I resorted to clapping, and I believe my eyes may have bulged.

"Oh, yes. My pain."

"Tell me about it."

"It hurts."

"Where?"

"The same places."

I again rested my forehead on a propping hand. She patted me on the arm this time. "Yes." She wriggled her shoulders. "I can't reach the spots. My back aches and keeps me awake nights."

I probed her back through her dress. "Tell me when I find the places."

"There, and there—ouch, that was sore."

Finally, something resembling a fact: pain and actual muscle soreness.

"For how long?"

"I think a year. Maybe two."

"I'll need to examine you more completely."

"It could be three."

I sat her on the end of the exam table and after a modicum of coaxing got her to strip to the waist and don a biblike patient gown, although her skinny arms allowed me only glimpses of withered breasts and the front of her chest. For the next three minutes—possibly five—we participated in a genuine medical experience.

She was made of bone, dainty muscles, and skin. I found half a dozen consistent points across her back that seemed genuinely tender. My stethoscope revealed a grade three over four apical murmur, which guaranteed that she had had rheumatic fever as a young person, but there was no sign of heart failure. All the while I was checking her, she huddled in an agony of modesty, and when I told her to dress again she said, "I *never* let Dr. Colleague do all that. A man shouldn't *ever* see a woman, especially if she is someone he knows. Not even a husband. Mother would *not* have allowed it."

I nearly wondered aloud how Minnie came to be, but I clung to silence. Instead, I picked up the Sears catalogue—her file—and scanned a few pages.

She said, "Dear, it seems so unfair that when you get older and can't do much else that you can't see to read. Someone should do something about that."

"Do you have trouble seeing?"

"I told you, I'm getting older."

"Um-hmm."

"When you're young, you take so much for granted."

"And your vision is . . . what, blurry?" I made notes, my attention parked in neutral.

"—and it's especially annoying when the lights go out."

"Lots of older people have trouble seeing after dark."

"Yesterday it was right after lunch, in broad daylight."

I finished my self-reminder notes and started for the door, had actually reached it before the sense of what she had said caught up with me. I came back and faced her.

"What did you just say?"

"When?"

"Something about when the lights go out."

"I don't like it. First one eye, then sometimes the other."

"Out? Like, do you lose all vision in the eye?"

"For a while, but then it comes back. Yesterday, while *General Hospital* was on, it lasted for several minutes."

"How many times has this happened?"

"Dear, I don't keep count."

"Do you have headaches?"

"Everyone has headaches. My father—"

I readied clapping hands. "What part of the head?"

She thought for a moment, then rubbed her temple. "It sort of throbs and gets sore."

I whirled and reached into the desk drawer for a laboratory requisition sheet. I escorted her to the hallway and located nurse Veronica.

Minnie Emerson said, "I don't think I'll take any lab tests. They prick you with needles and make you . . . you know, in a pan, and God knows what they do with that."

"It's important," I said.

"I think not."

I bent down until my face was near hers. "I *want* you to."

"Dr. Colleague never—"

I clapped my hands.

"Oh, dear. Veronica, this doctor is quite forceful, but not really brutish. Well, where do I have to go?"

Nurse Veronica's eyes were mostly whites, and her mouth hung open.

After Miss Emerson returned from her expedition to the hospital laboratory, I said, "I want you to return to see Dr. Colleague in one week for results of those tests we have to send away."

"I'll see, dear."

By mid-afternoon the lab reported her erythrocyte sedimentation rate (sed rate), and I called her at home. When she refused to return for admission to the hospital, I sent the county nurse, a persuasive lady named Samantha, to bring her back. Then I started her on the steroid prednisone.

Dr. Colleague was to return home that evening, so I scribbled a note to him, one not for the chart:

Thanks, pal. I learned a lesson today. Miss Minnie seems to have polymyalgia rheumatica, skinny little old lady with all the right signs and symptoms plus a sed rate of 126, as high as I've ever seen. I'll leave it for you to biopsy her temporal artery and nail it down. Proves that *anyone*, even our Miss Emerson, is entitled to a real disease.

Polymyalgia rheumatica: Also called giant cell arteritis, an aggressive and serious inflammatory disease of the arteries, affecting especially the back and the head. Usually found among the elderly, it can be fatal, yet it is easy to overlook. Transient loss of vision is a tip-off.

Potpourri

I ASSUME THAT MOST PEOPLE are basically decent; that, given a chance to know each other, differences will be small compared to compatibilities; that willingness to lend a helping hand is inborn. I hear occasionally of incidents in large cities where pleas for help are ignored by those nearby, and it is true that when I stroll down a busy street in Chicago or Pittsburgh or Minneapolis few of those I meet make eye contact or acknowledge my presence. A psychologist friend says this tendency is due to crowding, a need to preserve personal space.

Things are different in my Northpine. A walk of three blocks, the length of its main street, can take an hour. Not only do people see you, they expect to stop and chat. Publication of the local newspaper once a week is plenty, because all the news fit to print—and some that would require a heavy blue pencil—circulates immediately along the main street and beyond.

Barbara carried Northpine's friendly chattiness with her everywhere. On occasions when we ventured to the Twin Cities to see a play or to do some shopping, we would set out walking side by side, and within thirty seconds—I have timed it—I would be alone. Backtrack. Ah—there she was, in earnest conversation with someone she had never seen before.

An example: one day in Maplewood Mall, as we rested on one of the benches, a stranger, a tall, distinguished-looking, immaculately dressed, executive banker-type, approached. He stopped before us and stared at Barbara before plopping down next to her.

"My problem," he said, "is that our daughter is driving my wife and me up the wall. Now, we love her...."

I *swear* that opening is the absolute, unedited truth. Barbara spent half an hour ventilating the fellow. I, being as superfluous as the guy in the sunglasses booth across the way, settled back with a sigh. I never understood what it was about her: some aura visible only to a troubled soul?

.   .   .

A crow landed fifteen feet from where I stood, an inch-and-a-half-long crust of hard, dry bread in its beak. Head cocked, it studied me. I froze. It hopped to a small puddle, dropped the crust into the water, poked it around with its beak until saturated, then placed it on dry pavement. Holding the crust with one foot, the bird nibbled daintily.

I wonder: do we regularly underestimate the ingenuity of those around us? Even that of a crow?

.   .   .

Motor aphasia—loss of the ability to formulate words—usually from a stroke, is a frustrating handicap. Not uncommonly, the victims of such a brain insult understand what they hear and can conceptualize what they want to say. And, strangely, a phenomenon often accompanying this apparently complete wipe-out of vocabulary is retention of an astonishing assortment of profanity, words that would singe the hair of a buccaneer. I have heard a saintly nun and a former pastor—sweet little Aunt Bertha types—peel paint off walls. Even the most sequestered members of our race learn ribald expressions. Are we a species of closet cussers? Are such verdant words stored someplace where they can be unlocked by keys other than those of Broca's speech center, thereby managing to survive what is otherwise a total loss of vocabulary? I wonder.

. . .

For forty-six years I practiced medicine, and for forty-six years I was enslaved by communication electronics. Try to convince a doctor that there is charm in being constantly within grasp of a monster like a cell phone.

. . .

I interned at St. Luke's Hospital in Duluth, Minnesota, during the calendar year 1947. Interns and nurses keep the night watch in any large hospital, and it was our job to summon the appropriate attending physician when she or he was needed. Coping and communicating with sleepy doctors was one of those skills learned on the job: there is no med school course entitled Informing Grumpy Docs 101.

Some people sleep as though they have taken a two-by-four upside the head. Dr. D. was of this stuporous persuasion. We interns had a standard routine when summoning him for one of his deliveries: call at fifteen-minute intervals starting two hours before we really needed him.

I was on night duty when his patient, old Mr. Jonson, reached the end of the long trail. As was protocol, I telephoned Dr. D. to inform him of the death.

Dr. D. muttered, "That's good. Give him a shot of penicillin, and I'll see him in the morning."

. . .

A doctor takes for granted the mundane tools of the trade: a thermometer, a blood pressure cuff, a stethoscope. One day I left Northpine for Chippewa Lake in a frenzy of haste. When I unpacked at my schoolhouse office, I discovered that I had brought no stethoscope. A physician without one is like a fiddle player without a bow.

All afternoon my patients wondered what had snapped in that crazy *mookamoninini mushkikiwinini* (white medicine man) as he listened to their hearts with the pasteboard core from a roll of paper towels.

.   .   .

A consequence of surviving to the Octobers of life is having to say good-by to so many friends who don't.

.   .   .

Acute appendicitis is the most common emergency condition for which a nonspecialist like myself operated. But there are other conditions that mimic appendicitis so faithfully that it can be hard to diagnose for certain from "outside." In my day, sophisticated tests like the MRI and techniques like laparoscopy had not been invented. Occasionally one had to go inside the abdomen to check, because a missed infected appendix is lethal.

An inflamed embryonic remnant—an anomaly known as a Meckel's diverticulum—can present like appendicitis. A ruptured ectopic pregnancy in the right location can send the wrong signals. Crohn's Disease, a chronic but recurring bowel inflammation, can fool the most experienced surgeon.

Then there was Frannie V.

She came to the office with increasing pain in her right

lower quadrant, some nausea, a waning appetite, a slight elevation of her white blood cell count, and clinical signs of tenderness and tightness of the abdominal wall indicating acute inflammation of the peritoneal lining: peritonitis. I decided I needed to open her up to rule out appendicitis.

Frannie's appendix was normal. She had no Meckel's diverticulum, no chronic bowel inflammatory disease. But her peritoneum was obviously irritated. I searched with growing confusion. Then—

I found a two-inch-long, quarter-inch-diameter piece of bone wandering free in her abdominal cavity. A red spot in the wall of her small bowel, since sealed off, showed where the sharp-ended splinter had punctured it and been extruded.

We learned later that Frannie had eaten one of those canned chickens a day or two before her pain had begun. A drumstick loose in the belly: not your everyday malady. One chicken dang near got even.

. . .

So many deliveries occur in the middle of the night. A hoary medical joke holds that a pregnancy lasts nine months—to the minute. Assuming validity of the premise, one is left to wonder about those babies born during the lunch hour.

. . .

Drugs strong enough to nudge a bodily function toward a desired result often have what the profession calls "side effects." Shooting a fly on the wall with a twelve-gauge shotgun removes the beastie but, oh, those other "effects." Odd that ads for the latest pharmaceutical miracles don't stress this aspect of their products.

. . .

Touch, our most primitive sense, is also the most nurturing. The laying on of hands has survived from before biblical times. Yet a physician must ever monitor any impulse toward such common humanity as a hug, which these days can so easily become ammunition for a lawsuit.

During my forty-six years of practice, I hugged when it seemed to me the "medication" of choice: Ardith in her moment of atonement; tough, sometimes overbearing Officer Peterson on the night he coped with the death of his beloved daughter; twenty-six-year-old Alice Murdoch on the day I had to tell her that the numbness in her extremities was due to multiple sclerosis. I have not forgotten; I hope she remembers a moment of caring as well.

. . .

Our "office" on the Chippewa Lake Reservation, that sealed-off back entrance to the school building, allowed us to monitor the wonderful, universal sounds of children at play out in the surrounding yard. One day Barbara and I heard:

"My turn!"

"'Tain't, it's mine!"

"No fair! You hafta be the Indian an' I get to be the cowboy!"

. . .

Ancient Mary Squinteye needed medicine.

We had just loaded up the car for a return to Northpine after clinic at Chippewa Lake. I spied the arthritic old lady a hundred feet away, shuffling painfully toward us down a rocky path. I went to her and asked, "Do you need something, Mary?"

"Aspirin," she puffed.

"Wait here. I'll get it." I went back into the school, unlocked the medicine cabinet, poured a hundred aspirin tablets into a pill envelope, closed up, and returned to her.

"Here you are," I said.

"And some cough mix."

I trudged back to our schoolhouse office.

. . .

Martha M. was in my office for a prenatal exam. As she was leaving, I handed her a prescription for a vitamin and mineral supplement, and she laughed. When I cocked an eyebrow, she said, "My daughter Alice is seven now. I overheard her explaining to a comrade that if you want to have a baby, 'You just go to Dr. MacDonald an' he'll give you some "natal" pills that put a baby inside you somewhere until you have time to make clothes for it.'"

Tanya

TANYA WAS SIXTEEN the day I met her. She dragged into the examination room behind her mother, her lips a down-turned arc of defiance, her lids half-closed in a scowl. Eyes of a startling blue shade glanced everywhere but at Mother or me.

"Sit," her mother snapped.

She slumped onto one of the client chairs in that limber teenage way that seems to defy dictates of anatomy. She studied a fingernail chewed to a bloody quick and lifted it toward her mouth.

"Don't," barked Mother. Tanya rolled her eyes and sniffed.

I pulled my chair around to face them. "Who is the patient?" I asked, as if there were any question.

"I've had her to three other doctors and there isn't one of them give us any satisfaction," Mother said.

Ouch, set up already?

I sighed. "Why don't you tell me what's happening."

"She keeps having hysterical spells."

A quiet snort from the sullen youth. "Can you explain?" I asked Mother.

"If I could explain it, I wouldn't be here."

Aha. "Describe these 'hysterical' spells."

"She says she passes out."

"You mean you have not personally seen one of these episodes?"

Mother shook her head. "She acts okay to me, 'cept for her sass."

I turned to Tanya and leaned forward. "Can you describe how they are?"

She shrugged, attention on her ruined nails.

Mother erupted. "That's the way she is, tighter'n a locked safe, 'til she has one those spells, then she's weird for a while."

Tanya stabbed Mother with a glance like the thrust of a rapier. I stood up, directing my comments to Mother: "It's my policy to interview a young person in private. If you would wait in the outer office, I'll come for you when I'm ready."

Mother departed, radiating something less than approval. I sat facing Tanya at an oblique angle and brought my voice to a quiet level. "Are you here because you want to be or because your mother demanded it?"

She snorted robustly.

"Figured so," I said. "Next, we have to decide if your spending time here is worth the bother to you."

An even heftier snort.

"What's your name?"

She widened her eyes and stared pointedly at the chart on my desk.

"Do you pronounce it Tan-ya?" I asked.

"No! Tawn-ya!"

"I was right; you do have a nice voice. If *you* had decided to come here instead of being dragged along by your mother, what would you have wanted to discuss?"

She screwed her eyebrows and lips into a mocking question. "I have nothing to discuss!"

"Not even these spells I keep hearing about?"

"Them. They—they just happen."

"I'd be happy to listen to your version of events."

She shrugged.

I said, "Do you want to leave?"

Her eyebrows climbed a millimeter or two. "Can I?"

"Of course. This is *your* office visit, and you have the right to end it when you wish."

She bounded up and darted to the door. Hand on the knob, without turning around, she asked, "What would I tell Mom?"

"I'd leave that up to you," I said.

She pivoted slowly. "I could just walk out?"

It was my turn to shrug. She studied her feet. "What do you want to talk about?"

"Whatever you feel to be important."

She edged back to her chair and for the first time looked me squarely in the eye.

"I'm *not* hysterical," she said softly. I read entreaty on her face.

I leaned back. "For starters, why don't you just tell me about the so-called spells."

She pursed her lips, then relaxed on her chair. "I'll be just hanging with my friends and, like, the next thing I know, I'm on the ground or sprawled in a booth at the soda shop. It's sort of embarrassing."

Seizures? Convulsive or absence? I asked the standard questions: At what age did they begin? Any aura (premonition)? Ever a bitten tongue? Any loss of bladder or bowel control? ("Oh, ish," she said. "No!") Had anyone reported jerking or convulsions?

"No. Those other doctors asked about fits, made me get all wired up and electrified me. Mom blew a fuse at the cost, but they didn't show anything. I just—pass out."

"For how long?"

"Usually about, oh, ten seconds max."

"But you fall down?"

"Uh-huh."

Tanya's symptoms were not fitting her neatly into any syndrome I knew. Then—

She sat perched on the edge of her chair when abruptly, she—well, *imploded* is the word that popped into my head. Sudden pallor, eyes rolled up, joints completely loose. She slid toward the floor, and I caught her under the arms, her head flopping on a neck devoid of muscular tone. I lifted her onto the examination table beside us and checked her pulse. Pulse? There *was* no pulse! Frantic, I listened to her chest with a stethoscope: no *lub-dub* of a working heart. Just as I finished processing what the situation called for—CPR, and fast!—her heart flipped and began a steady beat.

Tanya opened her eyes. They looked around quizzically, and then she spied my anxious face above her. "Oh God," she said, "it happened again."

"And thankful I am, Tanya, that I was here to see it."

The entire event had taken no more than ten seconds.

By definition, rare medical conditions are, well, rare. An inane comment, yes, but one with implications. Always in the back of a country doctor's mind is the caveat that truly unusual conditions do pop up, even in a practice built on everyday problems. Rare or not, the doctor is expected to recognize what is happening and ask for help.

In time, consultants learned that Tanya had a congenital abnormality: electrical impulses required to keep her heart beating were periodically blocked, sending it into complete standstill for several seconds. Appropriate specialists fixed her up with an implanted pacemaker.

Tanya demonstrated a medical truism most graphically.

From the moment a heart ceases to pump blood around the body, the brain begins to shut down. Within three to five seconds, awareness goes, taking with it motor control. On such a narrow margin of safety does life depend. Yet so tough, so dependable is a heart that only in rare cases does the question even arise.

Tanya and I became comfortable with each other, and after she no longer had to live in fear of social disgrace—or even sudden death—we had a chance to consider the thorny issue of mothers relating to teenaged daughters during that period when independence struggles to try uncertain wings. A chance to talk to someone not burdened with being her parent; a doctor's oldest remedy, Elixir of Time; and the balm of maturation programmed into our very genes: these accumulated so that the last I saw of Tanya, she and Mother had become the kind of friends who seek each other out for lunch.

Requiem

THERE IS ONE PERSON to whom I owe the most profound apology.

It was in the second year of my practice. I cannot remember his name. I saw him only once; I did not see him alive. He was an infant, if nine months is still considered infancy. It was the middle of the night when I examined his body, in a shack in the far northern reaches of vast St. Louis County. Light seeped from a kerosene lamp. Somber family members, standing or sitting, watched.

"What happened?" I asked.

"He fell."

"How?"

"Out of bed."

"When?"

"Just before we sent someone to call you."

"And?"

"He fell and he cried and then—he quit."

He quit.

In 1949, society had not considered the possibility that family members—a father, a mother, siblings—might beat a child so badly that a vital organ would burst. I was a product of that society and its willful blindness. I know now, with every atom of my being, that I held in my hands that night the body of a bruised and scorned child, that I cradled it in hands dedicated to truth and healing. Instructed by ignorance, restrained by fear, unwilling to name the demons some members of our species can be, I agreed that a boy could die from falling fifteen inches onto the floor.

Nameless little boy child, hidden away in some equally obscure grave: your being, the example of your death, prodded me eventually into accepting the greater responsibility that goes with being a physician. I pray that your place in heaven is a special one.

Folk Medicine

FOLK REMEDIES have a long and sometimes speckled history. Foxglove yields digitalis, a mainstay remedy for a failing heart. Quinine to fight malaria comes from the bark of a tree, and a key ingredient in aspirin, salicylate, occurs in willow bark. Trial and observation awarded these and many more therapeutic agents to our ancestors. But searching the plant kingdom for useful drugs is a lottery, with more misses than hits. Brew up a concoction and human nature, through placebo effect, can conjure a response. Treatment and improvement may be wildly unrelated. Factor in some manufacturer's desire to profit, combine it with the sophistication of the advertising industry... be careful what you believe.

The doctor-patient relationship is imperiled when the physician must debunk some catchy new treatment based more on wishful thinking than on medical fact. Anson Kramer, owner of a local business, reported proudly that he had "cured" himself of some vague, self-diagnosed illness by paying a far-sighted entrepreneur for a chance to sit in an abandoned uranium mine. Or consider another chain of illogic: chelating agents combine with heavy metals, such as lead, arsenic, and mercury, allowing the body to excrete them; hardening of the arteries is characterized by the presence of calcium, which acts chemically as a metal; ergo, chelation should solve the problem. Not so. A doctor can understand a patient's intuitive leap of faith that if the process affects one variety of metal it surely must do as well at removing a similar element. It is harder to be charitable toward those who cynically profit from a frightened person's naiveté.

One of the largest schisms separating a scientist from one not trained in the discipline has to do with what can safely be considered proof. Is result A due to "treatment" B, or did dreaded coincidence take a hand? I have spent the equivalent of months of my life explaining the difference between hard scientific reproducible fact and testimonial evidence, like "Johnnie says treatment X cured him of some dread malaise, so, Doc, how come you won't give me the same?"

Trebor (BoB) Nosnah comes to mind.

Trebor was a bachelor. He lived to heck and gone out past Hardscrabble Road, making him a hermit in the eyes of many Northpiners. His hair style and attire reflected a bathing policy defined by whether or not he happened to fall into the Little Fork River while poaching walleyed pike. His name snagged attention, being a backwards rendition of Robert (BoB) Hanson. (Trebor was touchy about why he'd elected to write his name right to left. The time I asked him about it, he sputtered, "Dang it, Doc, BoB is BoB goin' either way!")

One day BoB poured boiling water on his arm: scalded the heck out of it. For several days he "treated" it at home in his shack, until it swelled to half again the size it was meant to be. Then he hitched a ride into town with logger Fabor Townsend.

That arm was ripe. A dirty brown granular material covered it, something other than sloughing skin and raging infection. I scratched my head. "What the heck *is* that stuff?"

Trebor glanced about conspiratorially. "Medicine, Doc."

"Trebor, I'm almost afraid to ask what you used, but I need to know."

"A secret. Been thinkin' I might cash in from it."

"I won't tell anyone."

"Well, see, like, Doc, you guys is all excited 'bout these here antibiotics, only they cost a man an arm and a leg. Figured how to save me some money."

"I hope that 'arm' reference isn't prophetic, Trebor."

"Come again?"

"Sorry. You were explaining."

"What I done, Doc—no tellin', now—I used my own anti-biotic. Heard that they come from a fungus, like, so I dosed 'er up good with puffball mushrooms. Hard to find enough those suckers this time of year." He beamed.

I sighed.

Question: how does one remove a heavy coat of puffball spores from a deep second-degree burn? Anyone?

ER, Northpine Style

M OST EMERGENCY ROOM calls that occur after midnight involve the following equation: alcohol + irresponsible behavior = blood and guts + an annoyed physician.

There are exceptions. Take the case of John Kangelmeier.

I received a telephone call at 3:00 AM. That part was usual. When I dragged myself into the emergency room, I found fourteen-year-old Johnny lying on the examination table and Boy Scout leader Bob French slouched beside it. "What's the problem?" I grumped.

John opened his hand, wincing. Two fishing lure tines, severed from their plug, were imbedded in the palm. I sighed and looked meaningfully at the wall clock.

Bob French said, "Sorry, Doc, but this happened out in the Boundary Waters Canoe Area Wilderness. We've been paddling and portaging for fourteen hours to get here. Kinda hard in the dark...."

Perspective.

·   ·   ·

Orthopedics, as related to trauma of the kind common in tourist country, intrigued me. So many medical situations involve diseases draped in obfuscation, but a broken bone is a broken bone. Obvious. Most of the fractures I saw were what we call "low-impact." Few caused by train wrecks, for example. Healing potential favorable. Over time I learned which injuries I could reasonably care for, and I discovered satisfaction in fixing them.

Three categories of fractures were most common. One was Little Old Lady Sightseeing Syndrome. There are few level places around Northpine, and all paths lead to vistas that even catch the eyes of locals. Little Old Lady skips down a slight rocky incline for a better view. Her foot slides on sand or a scattering of leaves, then her heel catches and momentum carries her body forward, causing a typical fracture-dislocation of the ankle. A couple of well-placed stainless-steel screws, and Little Old Lady is back together.

Or ski fractures. Proximity to a well-known ski hill provided hours of work for us there in Northpine. Most of the time what looks devastating on an x-ray—a spiral break of the tibia, the distal end of the fibula broken—heals well without the need for an operation.

Or loggers. Woods work used to be a very dangerous occupation. Not that it is one to be treated casually today, but machines like neighbor Ray Hahn's tree harvester and other variations have made felling a tree more predictable. A cardinal rule among loggers is "don't work alone." Even so, sometimes individual work must seem inescapable. Gil and Ed are two cases that come to mind.

Usually a tree falls in the direction selected by the cutter: away. Once in a while, however, it will slide back off its stump and overtake the guy who just felled it. One frigid day, Gil could not outrun a tree that did just that. He ended up with a broken leg, caught under a large tree trunk's many tons. Trapped. His power saw, dropped in the face of disaster, was off to one side. Gil stretched as far—as captor tree—would—allow—

He inched the saw toward him, held it up in the air while he yanked the starter cord, got it snarling again, and then, sitting there alone in the snow, cut the tree trunk on one side of his leg and then on the other. He rolled the freed piece of tree out of the way.

Next task: get to town. He scooted backwards on his buttocks to his pickup truck, pulled himself into its cab, and drove to the hospital. Good man, Gil.

And Ed: he also failed to outrun a tree that slid backwards off its stump. The heft of the large tree, its momentum, slammed into Ed's leg from the side. I have never seen a knee joint torn so completely asunder. I packed Ed's leg in ice, a means of slowing tissue metabolism in the presence of terrible injury. In Duluth, an orthopedist and a vascular surgeon awaited his arrival at the hospital. They saved his leg.

. . .

Cuts should be sutured, right? Well, sometimes. I was amazed by some of the wounds I was summoned to sanctify with stitches: a clean quarter-of-an-inch cut already sealed with serum, nature's glue, by the time its bearer arrives at the ER?

"But *Doctor*, you mean you aren't going to *stitch* it?"

Some of the largest "cuts" I have been called on to treat were distinctly *not* candidates for suturing. Like the time a young man fell into an asphalt paving unit and its auger gouged wounds deep into leg muscles, distributing tar along the way. Him we kept in protective isolation, the wounds covered with sterile saline packs until they healed by what used to be called "secondary intention." After all, nature has its own methods of healing: how do you think people got well before doctors were invented?

An encounter with a chainsaw, a frequent event in my Northpine, required its own special approach. The saw bites deep, the teeth carrying bark and wood chips far into the wound. Imagine what happens when one "kicks back," flying unexpectedly into the user's face. The individual, U-shaped blades of a saw chain, efficient at chipping out bits of wood, create a host of ragged tags of tissue in a person, leaving a wound mindful of an unzipped zipper. To sew up a cut of this type, thorough cleansing and debridement were necessary: wash out all the foreign material, then trim away the tags of skin and flesh—they do not survive anyhow, and dead tissue can provide fodder for nasty bacteria. Once the wound is converted into a nice straight edge, it can be sutured like any other.

Still, chain saws are ubiquitous around Northpine. Everyone owns one. Even me, although therein lies a story. I went to see my friend Dan with a mind to purchase one. He started to get the saw ready, stopped and stroked his chin, then turned to me and said, "Doc, I'm not going to sell you one. Sure as heck you'll cut off your leg, and then where would we be?" Bless you, Dan.

· · ·

During summers, a fishhook in the body tourist was a nearly daily event. Once removed, the hook was affixed to a felt-covered board by ER nurses Millie or Gladys or Vera. The board, cut in the form of a leering Pisces, was titled "Fish Who Caught People." A small tag identified the donor, the same idea as those pictures of some guy from Ohio standing on the dock beside a dead lake trout. We received much favorable comment from patients and visitors alike, with one exception: Ms. State Department of Health mandated its removal during one of her inspections, declaring it a dust catcher. Our man Clarence fixed a glass-covered frame to enclose it, so we felt we had won a moral victory of sorts. It wasn't the same, though.

The most unusual trophy on our board demands special comment. It was a lower plate. A dental plate, that is. See—to spare his feelings I'll call him Frenchie—Frenchie had been out fishing one day, and in the exuberance of a bass bite he swallowed the dang thing. It had wound its way through Frenchie's digestive system until reaching that last segment of bowel people seldom talk about in church. Or ever, for that matter. I dug it out, and for some reason Frenchie wouldn't take it home with him. I explained our policy of displaying trophies of piscatorial misadventure, and he said—actually in language not quite proper for a publication like this—that we could do whatever we wanted with it, so long as we didn't say whose it was. So, there's the story, folks. You won't tell, will you?

The Luck of the Chippewa

THE SIREN of an approaching ambulance plucks harp strings of my heritage: the part that reacts to a banshee's wail. The message: trouble imminent, death in the wings. Its summons means I must abandon whatever pursuit is at hand and focus my attention elsewhere.

The celebration known as Voyageur Rendezvous Days was in full swing at the Chippewa Lake reservation, a re-enactment of centuries-past annual meetings between the men who brought bales of fur to the shores of *Gitchigama* and those who exchanged them for trade goods that would buy the next year's harvest. A remarkable diversity of people attended the festivities: local Ojibwe; Native Americans from hundreds of miles away, from both the United States and Canada; and re-enactors of European descent, folks frolicking about in costumes purporting to be authentic, sleeping in mosquito-filled tents on Lake Superior's pebbly shore, throwing axes at targets, squalling on poorly tuned bagpipes (tuned bagpipes being, of course, an oxymoron), and eating food prepared with as little concern for hygiene as had been the vogue those two centuries before.

Our family had a special link to the event: my deceased first wife, Barbara, was one-half Indian and had grown up on the reservation, and our children are tribal members. These days, my present wife, Jackie, two of my children and their spouses, plus a number of good Northpine friends and I form a Celtic dance band. Each year as part of the festivities we play two square-dance sessions at the rebuilt fort.

Still, duty intrudes. I am on emergency call one August during Rendezvous Days.

A boy, a reservation local, about five or six, falls off a dock into Lake Superior but is not noticed immediately. Estimates of the length of time he was under water vary from ten minutes to fifteen, perhaps more. Then, through the crystal-clear water a youth spots him lying on the bottom. The young Indian man jumps into the lake, brings the boy up onto the dock, and begins resuscitation. Someone calls the reservation ambulance and then me at the hospital in Northpine, thirty-five miles away.

During the wait after receiving a message of doom, a thousand thoughts bombard me. I plan; I pace; I pray a little. What will arrive: A cold, dead body? Someone all right, the entire episode blown out of proportion? I prowl, peering from the emergency entrance, stepping outside to listen for a siren, waiting, waiting, waiting.

Then, I hear it. The nurses and I charge outdoors with our emergency room gurney, with oxygen, airways, and warming blankets.

The boy is alive but deeply comatose. He lies in what is called decerebrate posturing, arms extended stiffly, hands and forearms sharply internally rotated, head drawn back—all signs of severe brain dysfunction. He is already receiving oxygen from reservation EMT workers. I start an IV and call the Duluth trauma center to alert its staff. Back in the ER, I help transfer the boy to the gurney for the Northpine ambulance, which will take him the rest of the way.

Wait. The boy relaxes his arms, stirs, fights the airway.

Coughs! He demonstrates in textbook detail an upward spiral past deep narcosis, through awakening reflexes, to petulance at the tubes' discomfort. We decide not to send him to Duluth and instead put him to bed in the Northpine Hospital.

When I make rounds the next morning, the boy's bed is empty. My pulse leaps, and then I myself leap backward as a bronze torpedo roars out of the hall and into the room, a mother and grandmother puffing in its wake.

What had allowed the boy to stay under water for up to a quarter of an hour and then walk away as though nothing had happened? Hypothermia is a killer, yet, in the case of this boy, a savior. Lake Superior is *cold*. Full immersion in its icy arms plunged his core temperature to the point where metabolism slowed sharply and brain cells gained precious time. Additionally, in a second miracle, the cold must have caused instant laryngeal spasm, a complete blocking of the windpipe. Water inhaled into the lungs rapidly diffuses into the vascular system, diluting blood and overwhelming the heart, causing abrupt and fatal failure.

The luck of the Chippewa.

The Doctor's Family Was Involved

THE FAMILY OF AN ISOLATED COUNTRY DOCTOR was inevitably involved in the medical scene. I don't mean simply the disruptions of family life prompted by my always being on call. (I once figured out that I had been on emergency call—this on top of regular office hours—more than ten thousand nights of my life. Of my *family's* lives.) No, there was more.

In a medical office, filing—transferring dictated notes and reports to chart, then chart to file racks—was an ever-present chore, as mentally stimulating as counting grains of sand on a beach. As each of my six children reached an appropriate age, he or she was drafted into the role of file clerk. (Perhaps a factor in why none chose to follow in my footsteps?)

During the first fourteen years of my practice, we lived initially in an apartment built into the hospital, then in a house directly next door, one hundred feet away. Barbara, the only RN in sight for most of those years, was on call as completely as was I. Our children grew up as honorary staff members. Their playground was the hospital basement, its circling walkway their racetrack. Patients and nurses, maintenance men Bob and Leonard, launderers Sully and Madden, cooks Kelly, "Sammy," and Mrs. Massey, with her fabulous sweet rolls, cheerfully spoiled them. The trite phrase "second family" was valid.

For those first years in the woods, pre-trained paramedical

people were unavailable. Excursions to Duluth or Minneapolis in vain attempts to recruit nurses or x-ray and lab technicians invariably brought the response, "Oh no, too remote." We taught our own helpers, local women. As for esoterica like physiotherapy, dietetics, occupational therapy, a hospital social worker: I'd heard of such disciplines, but they were as out of reach as Kansas was to Dorothy while lost in Oz.

.   .   .

A physician should never treat a member of his own family, for the objectivity needed to diagnose or prescribe flies out the window if the patient is kin. Yet the directive "never" is subject to the whims of fate.

I received a call from the high school: student injured during physical education class. I climbed up onto the edge of the deep pads they used for gymnastics and peered over.

Daughter Pamela looked back at me sheepishly. She had landed awkwardly—we in Clan MacDonald are not gymnasts—sustaining crush fractures of three of her spinal vertebrae.

Doctor, you are it.

.   .   .

It was 1954. Eldest daughter Mary had turned five the week before. I came home that evening tired from a forty-patient day. We sat down to supper, Barbara across from me, four-month-old Bruce on the table in his *Adickinagen,* an Ojibwe infant carrier.

"Where's Mary?" I asked.

Barbara said, "She still doesn't feel well. Complains of a sore throat, aches and pains. I wish you'd look at her again."

I had checked her briefly that morning and had seen nothing remarkable. "Kids are always sick with something," I said. I put aside my napkin and went to Mary's bedroom.

"How's my girl?" I asked.

"My throat's so sore, Daddy."

She lay flat on her back, no pillow. I checked her temperature: ninety-nine point four, barely an issue. Throat normal in appearance. "It's probably a virus," I said, "and your throat isn't inflamed."

"That's not where my throat hurts," she said.

"Oh? Then where?"

She touched the back of her neck. I was suddenly all attention. When I slid my hand under her head and lifted it off the bed, she stiffened and her neck refused to bend.

"Don't, Daddy, that hurts."

Stiff neck—"nuchal rigidity" in the jargon of the trade—pain, don't-feel-good malaise: Mary had meningitis.

Doctor, you're it!

An obstetrical patient was in labor: I dared not leave the hospital to take Mary to Duluth, 165 miles distant. So, with Barbara forcing an "angry-cat arch" to Mary's back—"Mama, it hurts! Don't—" I performed the spinal tap necessary to diagnose meningitis.

The spinal fluid showed seventy-five or eighty white cells per cc, more than ten times the number in a normal tap. The cells proved to be lymphocytes, one of the body's cell lines that indicates a virus infection.

Mary had poliomyelitis.

It is difficult for young people today to understand the terror polio inspired during that era. Children were the most vulnerable. There was no cure, no real treatment. The famed Sister

Kenney method was aimed at reducing muscle spasms and at keeping joints and muscles limber during healing. But what about prevention? Vaccines were barely off the drawing board, scarce even for medical people. And no particular behavior, no quirk in lifestyle, made one susceptible. All were at the mercy of blind, indifferent fate.

I called Dr. X., my usual pediatric consultant in Duluth. "I'm in a terrible bind," I said, "an OB in labor, no one to cover."

"Does she have any bulbar signs, any breathing difficulties?"

"Actually, no paralysis at all."

"Well, RAM, you know even here we'd just watch her. Look, if any weakness develops, maybe by then you could bring her down."

We watched, Mom and Dad, Nurse Barbara and Dr. RAM. God was good: Mary recovered with only a barely detectable weakness in a few back muscles. Bruce developed no sign of the illness. In my practice, a few cases popped up here and there, erratic occurrence the rule. September's crisp days and frosty nights brought an end to fear. For that year.

.   .   .

It was 1957, the time 3:00 AM. Barbara was early for delivery but clearly in labor. I was unable to persuade the physician who had agreed to travel to Northpine Hospital to oversee the delivery that this was so; thus, daughter Jane arrived with me as the un-planned launcher. Lively from the beginning, she was fine.

But Barbara had always had an unusual platelet-related blood-clotting problem, and that business of objectivity arose. I did not do as exaggerated a job of repairing her episiotomy as her situation required, and she bled fiercely from the site, an almost unheard-of event. Three or four transfusions later we were all able to go to bed, I with my traditional new-father migraine attack.

The process of becoming a father is tough on a guy, even when he isn't the doctor of record. I'm not sure new mothers understand how deeply a man suffers....

Gotcha!

. . .

Fast-forward fifteen years. I had refused to buy a snowmobile, had in fact forbidden any of the kids to ride one. Predictably, such a directive begs to be subverted. One day Jane borrowed a friend's sled during noon recess and went for a ride. She came to a stop sign, hit the accelerator instead of the brake, and scooted directly into the path of a Peterbilt truck and trailer loaded with five or six cords of pulpwood. She rolled under the cab's wheels and ended up in the ditch beside the pile of scrap metal that had been the snow sled.

I was home for lunch when my friend Ray, our lab and x-ray technician, called from the hospital. "Come quick, RAM. It's—it's Jane."

Doctor, you're it!

I made a record trip. My route, past the mangled snowmobile, only increased my anxiety.

Jane ended up with a smashed pelvis and a knee torn asunder but, incomprehensibly, no other serious damage. After three operations, her knee still reminds her of what a Peterbilt can do.

Son Allan? I once had to replace his dislocated shoulder while he writhed on the living room floor. Son Bruce? There was that time his head and a thrown bat collided during a softball game. Objectivity, ha!

Doctor, you're it!

· · ·

The average child under the age of ten has three to four, even five or six infections each year. Most are respiratory, most viral. Nature's scheme requires this annoying state of affairs because there are literally hundreds of candidates lined up waiting to infect each kid. Viewing a virus as a lock demanding its own specific key and immunity as the needed key, the immune process becomes similar to the craft of a locksmith. At first he starts with a blank, which he spends some time figuring out how to cut. Nature (and our locksmith) can hang the result on a pegboard for future use. The next time that same lock (or infection) comes around, he (or one's immune system) can quickly cut a new key from the old master. Voila.

I earnestly tried to convince frazzled mothers that one of the more important functions of school was to gather together all the community's kids and have them share viruses. The curriculum could be Immunity 101. And 102. And 103. It was a good way to develop resistance: in fact, the only way for most infections.

It was a hard sell.

A consequence of having six kids is that one of them will contract the current model of viral infection at school and distribute it in-house. Usually its spread is a domino process, each kid getting the virus from a sibling until all have partaken. Problem is, about the time kid number one is well again and back at the old germ factory, a.k.a. school, a different brand of cold will have hatched, and—bingo—here we go again. Given that four or five annual cycles is standard, the average house-wife with any number of kids is likely busy much of the year wiping noses, doling out cough mix and acetaminophen for fever and aches, coping with irritable youngsters, and trying to get a moment's escape from her role as lion tamer.

Along about March one of those years, I walked into our happy home to be met with Barbara's rendition of "I've had it!" I explained about the locksmith, proud of my metaphor, how logical it was, even rather beautiful when you got to thinking about it, nature and—

Smack between the eyes, she hit me with, "Damn it, you're a doctor. *Do something!*"

This became our buzz phrase for those little-touted joys of being a parent.

.   .   .

I even took a turn at being my own patient. Searching my back for wood ticks one day, I found a dark mole over the left shoulder blade. My mentor, Dr. Ralph, whacked it off, and I sent it to a pathology laboratory in Duluth. The submittance form named me as referring doctor as well as patient, but Dr. Arthur missed the fact that the specimen was a hunk of me, so when he sent the report—"extremely malignant melanoma with a very poor prognosis"—I had no preparation. But then, how does one cushion a death sentence?

I underwent large-scale excision of the whole scapular area, including an axillary node dissection, followed by skin grafting. That, ladies, gives me real empathy for when a surgeon does the same to you as part of a breast amputation, and you experience the consequent painful swelling of the arm.

For twelve months Barbara, Mary, and I lived with the assumption that I would be dead by the same time the following year. Year one turned into year two. And then year three. Hope arose from its crypt, and we allowed ourselves to have our other kids.

My prognosticators proved to be wrong. Still, no single lesson in my medical education compares with being granted the terror of believing at age twenty-eight that I would never see twenty-nine. When I had to deliver to one of my patients that sledgehammer blow to hope and life, at least he or she knew that I understood. In an odd way, thank you, oh Fates.

Still, practicing alone in the woods for all those years—Doctor? Help? Please? Someone?

Heaven

I HAVE BEEN A FATHER to six wonderful children. Grown now, they have become, through the mysterious alchemy of maturation, friends. Some of them have themselves become parents. Jenna is one of my "grands."

Jenna had come to spend the day with Grandpa. She looked up at me with a six-year-old's eyes, the very definition of the word "trust," and said, "What is 'died,' Grandpa?"

"Why do you want to know?" I asked.

"My friend Rudy wasn't in school today, and Miss Hammerschmidt said he died."

Ah, Rudy Shotek. Dead of acute leukemia at age six.

"When will he be back to school?" Jenna asked.

"He won't be back."

She cocked her head. "Why?"

How to explain? At six, all of life is a mystery. "That's the nature of dying. It lasts forever." I recalled a story. "Remember the purple finch that flew into the window last summer?" Our picture window reflected a looking-glass land that seduced an occasional bird into trying its illusory depths. The finch had broken its neck with a rattling thump. Barbara told me what followed:

Jenna ran into the yard and returned with the bird cupped in her hands. Its head hung limply, eyes closed, feathers disheveled. Tears wet the girl's cheeks. "It won't fly, Grandma!" she said. Barbara explained that it was dead. "But why?"

"It's just not alive anymore."

"I want her to fly," Jenna said firmly.

"Honey, it can't; it won't."

"Then I'll take care of her until she does," Jenna said through her sniffles. Barbara explained about burying dead creatures, and Jenna asked, "Why?"

"Well, they decompose."

"What's that?"

"Bacteria grow—Ask your grandfather. I'll get a shovel."

Jenna shouted, "I'll do it! She's my bird!" She ran to a bank of sand, her play area, and with her toy shovel fashioned a sandy mound, complete with dandelion bloom.

Barbara waited until Jenna wandered off to explore our modest version of Pooh's Hundred Acre Woods before hurrying out to remove the finch to a more permanent grave. An hour later, Jenna burst through the back door, all flying colt shanks, blond hair a fuzzy halo in a beam of sunlight. She hollered, "Grandma, Grandma, my bird's gone! She—she—she already went to heaven."

I planted a kiss atop Jenna's head. "Mrs. Finch was dead."

"And she went to heaven."

"And now your friend Rudy is dead, from an illness. He won't ever be here again."

"Or talk?" she said. "He does in school, but the teacher makes him stop. Will someone bury him, like Mrs. Finch?"

When I asked her if she knew Jimmy Nelson, the town mortician, she shook her head. "He drives a school bus, too," I said.

She nodded, and her hair tickled my arm. "Amy says—He's so mean!"

"Jimmy mean? Why, I can't believe that."

She gripped the front of my shirt to look me squarely in the eye. "He is too! He makes everyone sit in their own seat and they can't even talk loud."

I hugged Jenna tight in my love and gratitude that it wasn't she whom Jimmy would have to bury.

Rudy Shotek had been a member of the neighborhood gang, Jenna's companions. She expected to attend the last earthly celebration of his existence, so we went to the visitation in Jimmy Nelson's funeral parlor. Jenna edged up to the casket uncertainly and asked, "When will he go to heaven?"

"He did when he died," I said.

"But he's still here!" I stumbled around an explanation: spirit, body, their differences.

She said, "When he goes, he'll be lonesome. I brought him a present." She dug in her little-girl purse and held out Procyon, her favorite toy. Lop-eared, one bead eye dangling, namesake of the Little Dog star, Procyon was a hand puppet of dubious pedigree. Jenna laid him in the casket beside Rudy's marble-white hand. "For him to play with when he gets to heaven," she said. She laid a scrap of paper next to Procyon. "I wrote a story, so he can read it." She looked up at me anxiously. "Do I need to put a stamp on it?"

Mute, I could only shake my head.

She smiled. "Now he's ready to go to heaven."

The Torch Has Been Passed

I CANNOT IMAGINE a career more fulfilling than mine. I enjoyed the unending variety a broad country practice affords, and I thrived on the opportunity to know my patients closely. I knew the answer to a question once posed to me: "Would you be missed, professionally, if you were not where you were?"

Is there a place in medicine today for a country doctor? Someone willing to help people through common colds, sprained ankles, hypertension, and diabetes, who finds satisfaction in ushering new life into the world? Someone at the same time unafraid to face the challenge of that rare "fascinoma," professional jargon for an unusual medical problem, when it shows up in the office? Someone not overwhelmed if at times she or he is the only doctor available? Willing to work longer and more unpredictable hours than a city cousin? Someone not aghast at the idea of making a house call? Comfortable with a role as parent-confessor to that person who most of all needs to talk, yet never forgetting that good intentions do not substitute for scientific knowledge or for well-honed skill? If one talks to the people I know best—colleagues and patients alike—the questions answer themselves with a resounding "yes."

During my years teaching for the Rural Physician Associate Program of the University of Minnesota Medical School, I met and worked one-on-one with more than two hundred third-year students. In a time when business performance appears to have captured the profession, when frustration and anxiety over matters medical are burgeoning, a citizen might rightly ask, "Where lie the hearts of the next generation of doctors?" When government and insurance companies threaten to wrest medical decision making from an on-the-spot doctor, what are the attitudes and aspirations of today's newest physicians? Cynical? Accepting of medicine as a business? Content to be time-clock punchers?

The young people with whom I had the privilege to work are still primarily and strongly motivated by a desire to help others. Forces driving new doctors into narrowing medical fields—the mystique of super specialization, doubt about mastering a broadly based core knowledge, apprehension about working alone, the burden of debt an average medical student acquires—have the effect of frightening off from rural practice all but the hardiest souls. Still, enough students choose country medicine that we who desire to live away from the city are not abandoned.

For making my life the joy and satisfaction it has been and for living with the restrictions imposed by an isolated solo practice, thank you family, thank you colleagues and other essential health-care workers, and, most especially, thank you patients, you who handed me your well being to hold in trust. I pray that we all live well and in peace.

Appendix

Careful planning was essential to the Cook County Cancer Screening Clinic's success. For more than twenty years, this task fell on the shoulders of county health nurse Rosemary Lamson, RN, MA. Blessed with unstinting energy and a talent for organization, she gracefully juggled all the factors that made the clinics work. Her master's thesis from the College of St. Scholastica (Duluth, Minnesota, 1991) records these achievements in detail.

The following citizens of Cook County, Minnesota, volunteered in the effort that came to be known as the Annual Cancer Screening Clinic, many of them year after year:

Sarah Allard, RN
Dorothy Almlie
Charlene Anderson
Gladys Anderson, LPN
Lou Anderson
Jan Baucher
Jan Beberg
Carol Berglund, LPN
Marilyn Berglund
Florence Bloomquist
Christie Buetow
Joy Carlson, LPN

Donna Clothier, RN
Community Action Programs
    (CAP) Office, Grand Portage
Shari Denniston, RN
Becky Deschampe
Melissa Ege, LPN
Ann Eliasen, RN
Verna Empey, LPN
Adair Erickson
Dorothy Esse
Vera Finn
Vera Flavell, RN

Cindy Gallea, RN

Mrs. David Gentzkow

Millie Gestel, RN

Ruth Gillis

Laurene Glader, RN

Rose Goble, LPN

Marie Hagen

June Hahn

Darla Halsa-Benrud, RN

Sue Hansen

Hildur Hedstrom

Ruth Hedstrom

Thelma Hedstrom

Amy Humphrey

Marsha Jackson, RN

Karen Jakala, RN

Vivian James

Esther Johnson, RN

Ethel Johnson

Grace Eileen Johnson, LPN

Mildred Johnson

Patricia Johnson

Margaret Joynes, RN

Alicia Kangas, RN

Virginia Killmer

Dorothy Krotz

Helen Kruse

Jerry Kruse

Rosemary Lamson, RN, MA

Bernice LeGarde

Jan Levin

Marie Lindemann, RN

Nancy Lindquist, RN

Sherrie Lindskog

Mrs. Richard Long

Virginia Lueth

Barbara MacDonald, RN

Gert Mahlberg

Marie Mark

Pat Martin, LPN

Dorothy (Donek) Mattson

Chris McClure, RN

Jan McKoon

Sophie Muehlberg

Marge Nelson

June Olsen

Mardel Otto, RN

Jean Peterson

Lillian Peterson

Thelma Peterson, LPN

Carol Quaife

Margaret Ranum, RN

Jean Roberts

Martha Rosbacka

Lois Sande, RN

Carol Seglem, RN

Rose Smith, RN

Lois Staples

Joseph Stevens

Sally Suck, RN

Mildred Swenson

Irene Thompson

June Thompson

Mildred Thoreson

Irma Toftey
Carol VanDoren
Linda VanDoren
Donna Viren, RN
Eleanor Waha
Harriet Walsh
Florence Weborg
Nelda Westerland

Dorothy Whipkey, RN
Beth White
Jean Williamson
4-H Club kids (for preparing
    envelopes)
Virgil Lindquist (supplies)
Mike Quaife (supplies)

The following physicians donated their time and talents for the examinations.

Physicians who lived and worked in Cook County for part or all of the twenty-seven years during which the clinics were held:

Barbara Bank, MD
Edie Broschat, MD
Thomas Clifford, MD
Bruce Dahlman, MD
Michael Debevec, MD
Robert Fish, MD
William Gallea, MD
David Hilfiker, MD
Dennis Kaufman, MD
Roger Lienke, MD
Roger MacDonald, MD
Ingrid Nisswandt, MD
Nancy Olsen, MD

Stephen Park, MD
Remi Pizzaro, MD
Peter Sapin, MD
Carl Sjoding, MD
Wallace Smith, MD
Sandy Stover, MD
Paul Terrill, MD
David Vesall, MD
Karen Virchota, MD
Carl Wall, MD
John Wilson, MD
John Wood, MD

Physicians who lived outside Cook County and who volunteered to work in the clinics free of payment, several for many years in a row:

Charles Bagley, MD

Elizabeth Bagley, MD

Charles Barbee, MD

Philip Bray, MD

Warren Brooker, MD

J. R. Creps, MD

Philip F. Eckman, MD

Philip L. Eckman, MD

Barbara Elliot, PHD

Dr. Erickson, MD

Mac Fifield, MD

Glen Holt, MD

Wayne Jarvis, MD

Franklin Johnson, MD

Nina Kastraba, MD

Ted Kubista, MD

Robert LaBree, MD

Janet Lindquist, MD

John Mathers, MD

Brian Meyers, MD

James Monge, MD

Dr. B. Monson, MD

Marvin Nevonen, MD

Dr. Owens, MD

Edward Ryan, MD

Dr. Sebastian, MD

Thomas Stolee, MD

Kenneth Storsteen, MD

Donald Swenson, MD

William Turner, MD

Paul VanRyzen, MD

Jack Wall, MD

Arthur Wells, MD

Thomas Wiig, MD

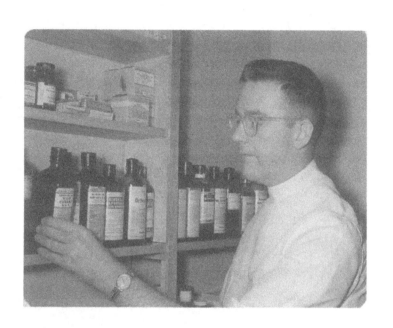

A Country Doctor's Chronicle was designed and set in type by Chris Long at Mighty Media, Minneapolis. The typefaces are Vendetta and Triplex Italic, both designed by John Downer. Printed by Maple-Vail Book Manufacturing Group.

Printed in the USA
CPSIA information can be obtained
at www.ICGtesting.com
JSHW022336140824
68134JS00019B/1513

9 781681 340234